3.16.79

inside
weight training
for women

**doris barrilleaux
and
jim murray**

cbi **Contemporary Books, Inc.**
Chicago

Library of Congress Cataloging in Publication Data

Barrilleaux, Doris.
    Inside weight training for women.

    Bibliography: p.
    1. Weight lifting.   2. Exercise for women.
I. Murray, Jim, joint author.   II. Title.
GV546.B36   1978   796.4'1   78-8105
ISBN 0-8092-7501-5
ISBN 0-8092-7500-7 pbk.

Photographs by Dick Falcon

Copyright © 1978 by Doris Barrilleaux and Jim Murray
All rights reserved
Published by Contemporary Books, Inc.
180 North Michigan Avenue, Chicago, Illinois 60601
Manufactured in the United States of America
Library of Congress Catalog Card Number: 78-8105
International Standard Book Number: 0-8092-7501-5 (cloth)
                                    0-8092-7500-7 (paper)

Published simultaneously in Canada by
Beaverbooks
953 Dillingham Road
Pickering, Ontario L1W 1Z7
Canada

contents

Acknowledgments   v

Introduction   vii

1   The Basic Program   1

2   Special Programs   19

3   When Overweight is the Problem   41

4   For the Fortunate Few Who Need to Gain Weight   47

5   Individualizing an Exercise Program   51

6   Nutrition and Weight Training   57

7   Strength and the Female Athlete   61

Index   67

acknowledgments

A number of people have helped us greatly in preparing this book. Dick Falcon, the photographer, worked beyond the call of duty to take the pictures in several sessions and then put in hours in an unusually cold darkroom making the prints. (Who could have anticipated that it would be cold in Florida, even in the winter!) And the models got more exercise than they bargained for in the outdoor sessions. Joyce Weir, Cindy Henning, Linda Carpenter, and Anne Leto hoisted barbells and dumbbells for hours, waiting for the sun to break through the clouds. (The sun is supposed to shine all the time in Florida!) Hector and Elisa were kind enough to allow us to take pictures in their beautifully appointed and superbly equipped Tampa health club, where the girls work out. And we were fortunate to have Jane Murray retype the manuscript, since her experience at the Bucks Fitness Center enabled her to check the instruction as well as tidy up the pages.

Doris Barrilleaux
Jim Murray

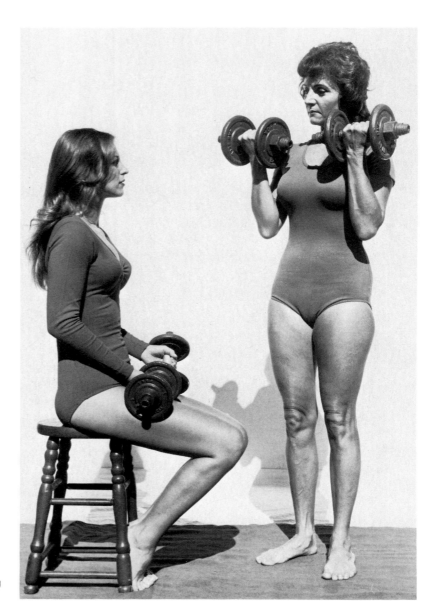

Doris Barrilleaux (standing) shows
Anne Leto how to do curls for upper
arm toning. Due to hormonal
differences, this exercise builds
biceps size for men, but firms the
upper arms of women without adding
significant muscle mass,

introduction

Weight training for women—does it make you think of burly Eastern Europeans heaving shotputs or Tugboat Annie types arm-wrestling the bartender? If it does, it shouldn't. Try instead the mental image of Marilyn Monroe and Tina Louise at their curvaceous best. Both film stars had learned something that was generally a well kept secret a couple of decades ago: weight training does not make normal women look like men. It makes them more shapely, but definitely in the feminine mold.

The reason Marilyn Monroe and Tina Louise didn't develop bulging muscles as a result of their weight training is that they were normal women with a full complement of female hormones, the biological controls that separate the girls from the boys.

The positive benefits of weight training for women have been confirmed by many more examples than a few film stars. Margaret Court, the Australian tennis star, reports that she trained with weights for years with no adverse effect on her appearance and positive benefits for her tennis game. In an interview with Mary Daniels, of the *Chicago Tribune* news and feature service, Ms. Court cited Jack Wilmore, an exercise physiologist at the University of California, "who has been putting hundreds of coeds through weight training for several years. He has discovered that when men and women lift weights side by side, the men develop muscles and the women develop shapely figures."

It is well known by physiologists that the larger muscles developed by men result from the male hormone testosterone. Actually, men and women secrete both testosterone and the female hormone, estrogen; but in the normal male, testosterone predominates and in the normal female, estrogen predominates.

In addition to hormonal differences, both men and women have mixtures of three body types, or somatotypes. These are *endormorphy,* in which roundness and softness predominate; *mesomorphy,* in which muscle and bone predominate; and *ectomorphy,* in which thinness and fragility predominate.

Women tend to be more endomorphic than men, which reinforces the tendency of female hormones to produce wider hips relative to shoulders. Occasionally, however, a woman will have a strong mesomorphic component in her makeup, which results in her being huskier, in a solid sort of way, than most women. A mesomorphic woman will have relatively broad shoulders for a woman but will still not become as broad-shouldered and strong in the upper body as a man. She may develop leg strength comparable to men of her own size, however, except for very strong men who compete in weight lifting and other vigorous sports.

As long as a woman has a normal complement of female hormones, she can always look appealingly feminine, with curves in the proper places. And exercise will help mold all kinds of bodies into improved appearance, whether they are predominantly endomorphic, mesomorphic, or ectomorphic.

Some of the best examples of the appearance-improving effects of weight training for women were models and actresses who exercised under the guidance of George Bruce at his California gym. Among the major beauty queen awards collected by his pupils were Miss USA of 1956, won by Paulette Nelson; Miss USA of 1962–63, won by Amedee Chabot; and Miss California of 1962–63, won by Marilyn Tindall. Ms. Tindall was also third runner-up in the U. S. division of the 1962 Miss Universe Pageant.

But even more important than the cosmetic effects of weight training for women, we believe, are the improved confidence and sense of well-being that this form of exercise imparts. Total physical fitness calls for activities that produce cardiorespiratory endurance—heart, lungs, and circulatory system—and strength.

Strength is often played down as a contributor to fitness, but well-toned muscles do much more than maintain pleasing body contours. If your legs never overcome any more resistance than moving your body around, merely moving your body around can be a strain. If your arms never encounter any more resistance than lifting a handbag or a sack of groceries, these everyday tasks can be fatiguing. But if you practice a few knee bends with additional weight in your hands or on your shoulders, and exercise your arms with dumbbells three times a week, the added strength you will build will make carrying your own weight and performing ordinary chores that much easier.

As Dr. Lawrence E. Lamb has pointed out in *The Health Letter* (Box 326, San Antonio, Texas), "a woman can tighten up her muscles and have attractive feminine curves with good strength (by practicing weight training) without fearing the development of what is classified as a more masculine physique."

Dr. Lamb notes that maintaining lean muscle mass helps prevent obesity. This is because "Fat tissue does not use as many calories as muscle tissue at rest." Dr. Lamb cites studies by Ancel Keys and his associates showing that "the decrease in use of calories at rest (basal metabolism) in different age groups was related to the change in muscle mass, not age." Dr. Lamb of course recommends that anyone in doubt about her ability to exercise should get clearance from her physician, but believes that "Most healthy people can benefit from a sensible weight training program."

FOR ADDITIONAL INFORMATION

This book provides a thorough summary of information and instruction on the use of weight training for women, but current articles and additional sources of instruction, such as advertisements for courses developed specifically for women, can be found in a number of publications. For example, *Strength & Health* magazine, P. O. Box 1707, York, Pennsylvania, 17405, includes a regular department "For Women Only" and publishes practical instruction in Vera Christensen's "To The Ladies" column. *Iron Man* magazine, 512 Black Hills Avenue, Alliance, Nebraska, 69301, publishes articles on women who train with weights.

Other magazines that publish articles or brief items on weight training for women include *Muscle Builder/Power*, 21100 Erwin Street, Woodland Hills, California, 91364; *Muscle Training Illustrated*, 1665 Utica Avenue, Brooklyn, New York, 11234; *Muscle Magazine International*, Unit One, 270 Rutherford Road, Brampton, Ontario, Canada; *Muscular Development*, P. O. Box 1707, York, Pennsylvania, 7405; and *Muscle Digest*, 1234 South Garfield Avenue, Alhambra, California 91801.

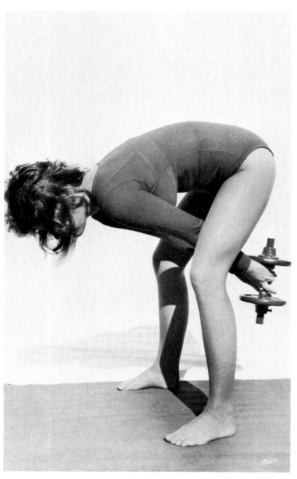

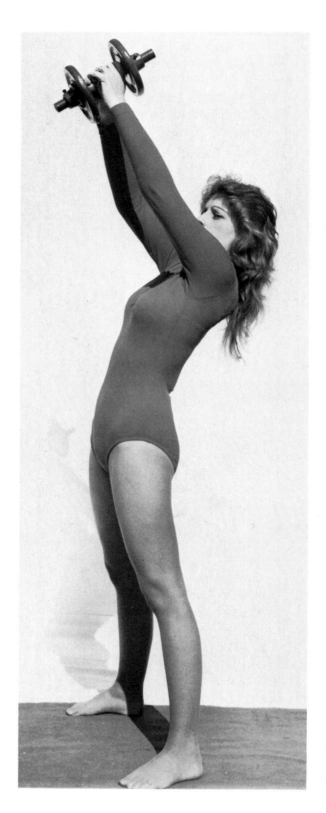

Linda Carpenter demonstrates the dumbbell swing, an effective warm-up exercise that involves all the muscles of the body. The exercise should be done smoothly, with control, allowing the knees to bend in order to take strain off the back.

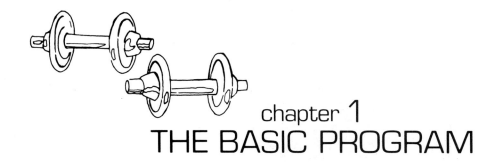

chapter 1
THE BASIC PROGRAM

For women with no special figure problems, handicaps, or athletic training ambitions, a very basic program will improve physical fitness and appearance if followed three days per week. The program is intended to tone, strengthen, and improve the shape of every part of the body.

WARM UP FIRST

Before beginning exercises for specific body parts, it's a good idea to prepare your muscles for the work by doing a few loosening-up movements. Reach overhead and bend to touch the floor, allowing your knees to bend slightly. Repeat this reach and bend several times. Then make it more difficult by holding a small dumbbell with both hands. Raise the dumbbell overhead and then swing it smoothly down and back between your legs. Without stopping, swing it back overhead and repeat five to ten times. This dumbbell swing is a movement similar to chopping wood and is an excellent overall warm-up exercise.

The exercises in the basic program are arranged so they will contribute to warming up your body for the more difficult exercises in the routine.

SIT-UPS FOR THE ABDOMEN

The first exercise, the sit-up, is an abdominal strengthener and trimmer, but it also stretches and loosens up the entire torso. You should learn to do sit-ups properly for best results. If you simply assume the correct position and mechanically do the sit-ups it will help, but the exercise is much more effective if you *think* about contracting your abdomen and pulling your waist in. Here's how: Lie supine (on your back) and draw up your knees so your legs are bent as shown in the illustration. Either tuck your feet under a piece of furniture, have them held down by a training partner, or anchor them under a pad or strap on a sit-up board. At first you may have to reach forward with your arms to help you sit up. Later you can do the exercise with arms folded. When you get your abdominal muscles in

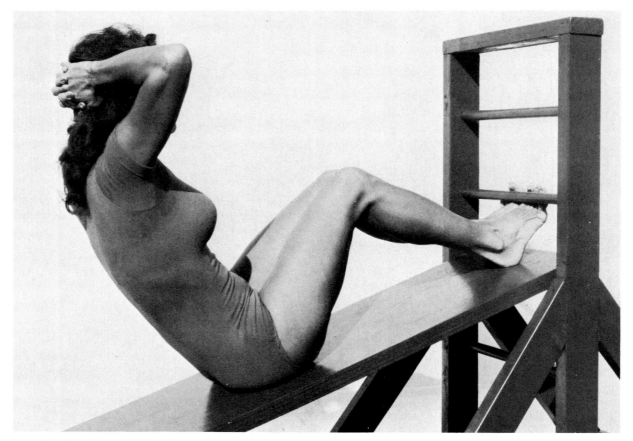

Doris Barrilleaux shows how to do an advanced sit-up, using an incline to add to the difficulty. Beginners should do sit-ups on a flat surface and may reach forward to help get up until the abdominal muscles gain strength.

good condition, you can do the exercise with hands clasped behind your neck, and ultimately, you may want to hold a small weight behind your neck.

Once you're in the supine position, with knees bent and feet anchored, take a breath and then *exhale,* consciously pulling your abdomen in and tilting your pelvis upward as you roll up into a sitting position.

As soon as you're up and leaning forward slightly, return to the supine position and inhale. Exhale before you sit up again. If you get out of breath doing sit-ups, pause in the down position and breathe a few times until you feel ready to continue to exercise. But do each sit-up after a deliberate inhalation and exhalation that enables you to pull your waistline in as you sit up.

Try to do ten repetition sit-ups without stopping to rest. If you can't do ten, do as many as you can, rest awhile, and then do more until you reach a total of ten. Ten is enough to do for the first week or two, but if you can do ten easily after two weeks, increase to 15 or 20. Fifty is not too many sit-ups to do if they're easy for you; but if you're trying for muscle tone rather than reducing, it will do you more good to keep the repetitions in the ten to 20 range and hold a small weight (two-and-one-half to five pounds) behind your head than to do large numbers of sit-ups. If you get to the point where you can sit up 20 times with a ten-pound weight behind your head, you should have exceptionally well-toned abdominal muscles and should not need to work any harder on the exercise. In fact, 20 sit-ups with a

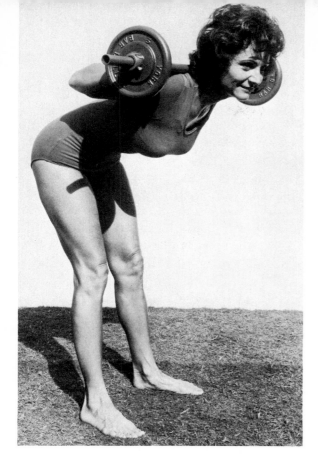

When doing forward bends (the good-morning exercise) to strengthen the back muscles, move smoothly, with control, and allow the knees to unlock (to bend slightly) in order to avoid undue strain.

five-pound weight represents excellent abdominal strength and muscle tone.

Don't forget, as you do sit-ups, to strive for the correct *feel* of the exercise. As you exhale, tilt your pelvis upward, and begin to raise your head and shoulders, you should feel your abdominal muscles tightening over visceral organs that are being pulled down by gravity. That sensation of taut rubber bands pulling up and down all along your tummy means that you are getting results, that you are developing a natural girdle of muscle to hold your organs properly in place without sagging.

FORWARD BENDS FOR THE LOWER BACK

You have your choice of either of two exercises for low-back muscle tone. You can either hold a light barbell across your shoulders, or hold a light barbell or two dumbbells in your hands while doing forward bends. If you hold the bar across your shoulders, it's called the good-morning exercise (like a polite bow) and

if you hold weight(s) in your hands, it's called the stiff-legged dead lift. Except that we don't want you to keep your legs straight. Instead, bend your knees very slightly and then bend forward smoothly and carefully until you feel a comfortable stretch in your lower back. Return to a standing position and repeat for a total of ten forward bends.

If you do the exercise holding a barbell or dumbbells in your hands, lean well back and shrug your shoulders back as you straighten. You can try to do this as you straighten from the good-morning exercise too, but it's not as easy to shrug your shoulders with the bar across them as it is when it's hanging at straight arms.

It is very important to strengthen the lower back and abdomen, which is the effect of the first two basic exercises. But be cautious in doing a forward bending movement. If you are a person who is prone to low-back strains, be especially cautious. If you know you have a low-back problem, you may want to substi-

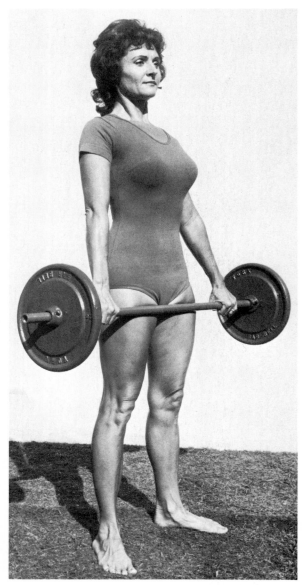

Note that Doris Barrilleaux fully straightens, with shoulders back, at the completion of a deadweight lift. Doris, pictured at age 46, has been married 30 years, has five children and five grandchildren. She has been practicing and teaching weight training since her teens.

tute the hyperextension exercise (described in Chapter 2, Special Problems) for a forward bend movement.

You don't need much weight resistance for the forward bending movements. An unloaded barbell handle or a pair of five-pound dumbbells is plenty of weight to start with. If the exercise is easy for you

and you feel that ten repetitions is not producing enough results with ten to 15 pounds (the weight of an average unloaded exercise bar), you can increase the resistance gradually, five pounds at a time (two-and-one-half pounds on each end of a barbell) until you reach a weight that seems adequate. If you're ambitious, you may work up gradually to a total weight of 30 to 50 pounds, but unless you're building strength for a competitive sport, there is no need to go to any heavier weights than these.

PRESS FOR SHOULDERS, ARMS, AND UPPER BACK

Our next three exercises are for the arms and shoulders. First is the press overhead with dumbbells or a barbell. In this one, you hold the weight(s) at your shoulders and push it (them) straight up overhead until your elbows are locked. 'Unlock them immediately, lower the weight(s) to shoulder height, and repeat ten times in succession.

If you're using a barbell, hold it with an overhand grip (knuckles away when you pick it up). If you're using dumbbells, turn them so they point out from your ears, palms forward as you press. Space your hands slightly wider than your shoulders on a bar. Start with dumbbells at the outer edge of your shoulders.

Take a breath before pushing the weight(s) upward, exhale as your arms straighten, and inhale as you lower the weight(s) for the next repetition.

Incidentally, when lifting the weight(s) to your shoulders for the press, keep your back flat or slightly arched (the opposite of rounded) and bend your knees as you raise the barbell or dumbbells from the floor. Whenever you lift *anything* from below the waist level (except when deliberately doing a forward bend exercise), you should bend your knees and crouch with your back flat or slightly arched.

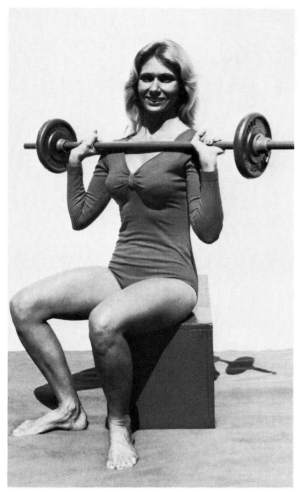 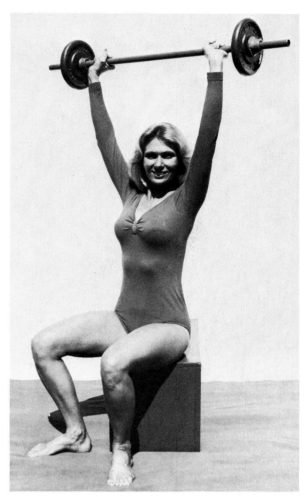

Joyce Weir demonstrates the barbell press while seated. The exercise is easier to do while standing. Joyce, pictured at age 32, has two children.

Your hip joints should be somewhat lower than your shoulder joints and your back should *not* round when you lift from the floor.

When pressing weights overhead, try to keep your upper back flat and your elbows out to the sides. You can do repetitons of this exercise for additional back-flattening effect, by lowering the bar to touch your shoulders behind your neck. Don't try to handle heavy weights in this exercise, but the weight should be enough that you feel some muscle toning effect with ten repetitions. If the weight becomes too light, add two-and-one-half pounds to each end of the barbell. Most women will not want to go much beyond a total of 20 to 30 pounds of resistance, but be governed by how you feel. A strong woman might press 40 or 50 pounds for ten repetitions, but there is no need to increase the weight beyond an amount that produces a sensation of pleasant muscular fatigue. Leave the heavy weights and hard iron-pumping for men.

CURLS FOR THE FRONT OF THE ARMS

To tone the front of your arms (the biceps area), hold a barbell across your thighs with an *under*hand grip (thumbs outward) and your hands spaced shoulder

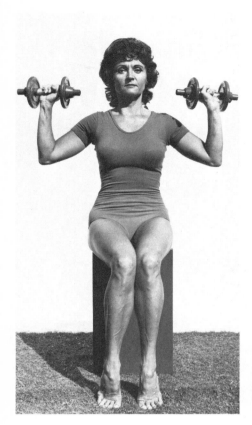

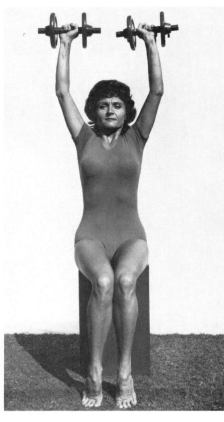

Dumbbell presses are more difficult than barbell presses because of the need to control two separate weights, and they are more difficult to do seated than standing.

Curls can be done in either a seated or standing position. The palms are turned upward as the weights are raised to the shoulders. The exercise can also be done with a barbell.

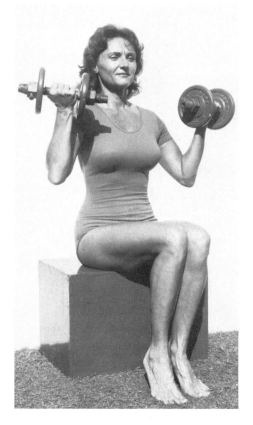

width. Keeping your upper arms at your sides and, standing straight, bend your arms so the barbell travels in an arc to your throat (this is called curling). Nothing should be moving except your arms from the elbows to hands. Inhale, curl the weight, exhale, lower the weight, and repeat ten times in succession (ten repetitions, or reps).

If you're using dumbbells, hold them in a natural position at your sides, knuckles out, but turn your palms up as you curl the dumbbells to your shoulders.

The curl strengthens and firms the biceps area (on men, because of their different hormones, it also builds arm size).

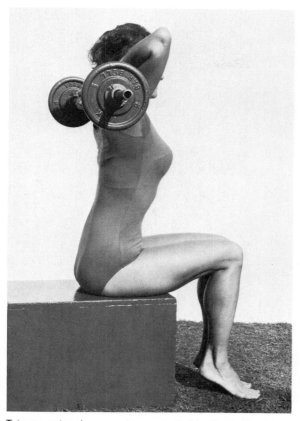 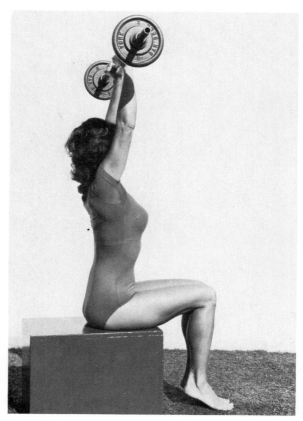

Triceps extensions, as demonstrated by Doris Barrilleaux, are unexcelled for firming the backs of the arms where many women tend to become flabby.

TRICEPS EXTENSIONS FOR THE BACKS OF THE ARMS

The overhead press helps tone the backs of the arms, but this becomes a problem area for many women, and it's a good idea to do a very direct exercise for the triceps, as the muscles in the back of the arm are called. The exercise can be done in several ways; here's one of the best:

Hold a light barbell with a narrow, overhand grip or a single dumbbell with both hands. Lift the weight straight up overhead. Then, keeping your upper arms pointing straight up, allow your forearms to bend until your hands travel in an arc to the back of your neck. Immediately force the weight back overhead, keeping your elbows pointing up and moving nothing but your forearms.

Do ten reps of the triceps extension. If you do it right there will be a pronounced stretching and tightening of the backs of your arms as you lower and raise the weight, and you will feel a soreness in the area for a day or two after the first time you try the exercise.

TWISTS TO TRIM THE SIDES

An excellent exercise to tone and trim the sides of the waist is done holding an unloaded barbell handle or a broomstick across your shoulders, arms stretched out along the bar or stick. In a seated position with feet locked against the object you are seated on, alternately twist (turn) your body around as far as possible to one side and then the other.

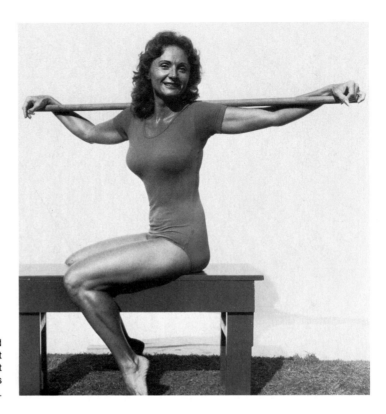

Twisting, as shown in the photo, tightens and slims the sides of the waist and the upper part of the hips. The legs should be kept tight against the bench to anchor the hips and focus the action on the sides.

Keep your legs firmly in place to anchor your hips and focus the effect of the twisting on the sides of your waist above the hips. Start with ten to 20 twists to each side and gradually work up to higher repetitions by adding one or two each time you exercise. If you have no special waistline problems, a total of 50 (25 each way) may be enough, but don't hesitate to go on to 60, 80, or 100 if you think you need the work.

SQUATS FOR TRIM AND SHAPELY THIGHS
Squats (knee bends) with weights are unexcelled for toning all the muscles of the upper legs and hips. This toning effect contributes to shapeliness. The exercise can be done while holding a barbell across the back of the shoulders or while holding two dumbbells at shoulder level.

With the weight at the shoulders, stand with feet about hip width apart, toes pointing slightly outward. Take a breath high in your chest and, holding your

abdomen in and back slightly arched, sink with controlled muscular effort until your thighs are level with the floor. Rise immediately, exhaling as you straighten your legs. Inhale and repeat for a total of ten squats.

If you have trouble keeping your heels on the floor and/or keeping your back arched as you reach the low position, try placing a one-inch thick board under your heels. If you continue to have trouble holding the correct position, try a thicker board under your heels.

Squats stretch muscles in your legs that aren't used to being stretched, so don't overdo the first couple of workouts. Don't be surprised if you feel muscle soreness for a day or two after your first couple of exercise sessions, especially along the inner parts of your thighs. The fact that you do feel the soreness should be encouraging, however, for you will realize that you have activated a portion of your legs that often is underdeveloped

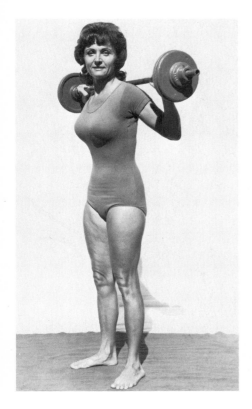 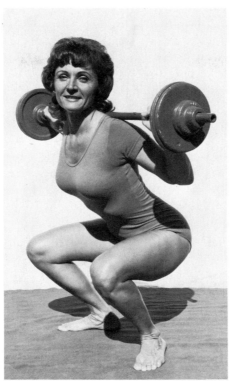

Squats with a weight should be done exactly as Doris Barrilleaux shows in the photos, with the back held flat or slightly arched. It is not necessary to go any lower than shown.

on women, causing a hollow appearance of the inner thighs.

Start with an amount of weight that is fairly easy to use for ten repetitions, but try to add five pounds every week or so until you feel you are using enough to make it reasonably difficult to complete ten repetitions. Twenty to 50 pounds is enough to strive for, but if 50 feels too easy, don't hesitate to move on to heavier weights. As long as you can do ten repetitions properly, in good position, you are not using too much weight. There is no reason an average-size woman in good condition shouldn't do squats with 75 to 100 pounds if she's ambitious and has the aptitude for it. Many topflight women athletes do squats with 200 pounds and more. If you do become ambitious and

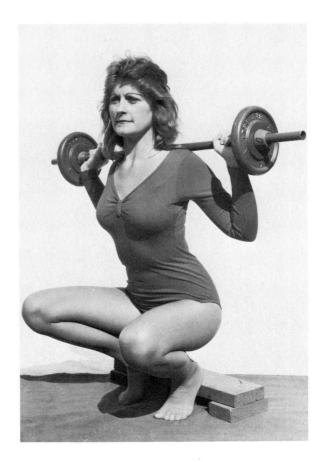

Linda Carpenter demonstrates a very deep squat with a thick elevation under the heels. Most people will not need to brace their heels this high or squat so low. This method of performance focuses the effort on the lower thigh, near the knee.

want to use heavy weights, however, be sure to have one or two people standing by to help if you get stuck in the down position.

PULLOVER FOR POSTURE AND CHEST EXPANSION

The next exercise, the pullover, should be done after squats because if you've done them with proper concentration on making the effort, you should be somewhat out of breath. The pullover is a deep-breathing exercise and will help you recover. The main purpose of the pullover is to stretch the rib cage, increasing vital capacity and improving posture.

Do the pullover like this: Hold a light weight (two very light dumbbells, a single dumbbell held in both hands, or a barbell plate on a short piece of pipe, held with one hand on each side of the plate with an overhand grip) and lie supine (face up) on the floor or—preferably—on a bench. Hold the weight straight up over your chest and then lower it smoothly in an arc behind your head, inhaling as the weight

goes down. Time your inhalation so your lungs are full just before your arms reach full stretch. Without pausing, pull the weight back up over your chest, exhaling. You may bend your elbows slightly at the start of the exercise; but if you do, hold the same bend throughout the movement. If you can do the exercise with arms straight, the stretching effect will be better. Lower the weight and repeat, concentrating on inhaling with stretch on the way down, exhaling on the way up, for ten repetitions. Five to 15 pounds is plenty of weight. The resistance is used only to help you stretch and to use up some of the oxygen you're taking in, to help prevent hyperventilation (an excess of oxygen and a deficit of carbon dioxide in the body from overbreathing).

STRAIGHT-LEG KICKS, PRONE

The next two exercises are for the problem areas of the hips and upper thighs that plague so many women. It isn't necessary to use weight resistance with these exercises, but they can be made more

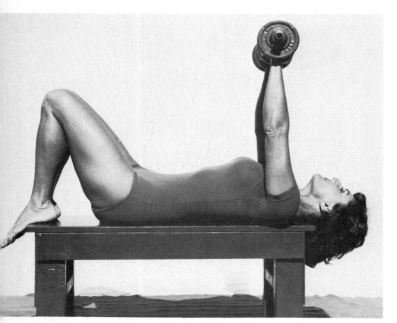
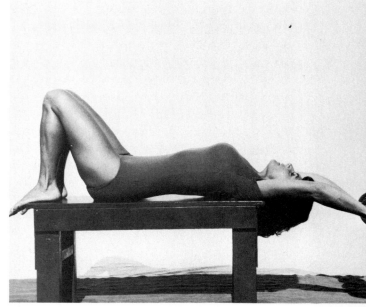

This is the range of motion needed in the pullover to fully stretch the rib cage and pull in the abdomen.

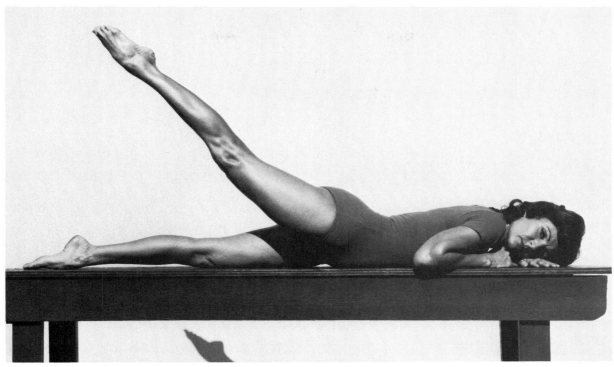

Straight-leg back kicks in the prone position tighten and firm the backs of the hips.

effective by wearing an ankle weight or a metal health sandal, sold via mail order by such companies as the York Barbell Company (Pennsylvania) and the Weider Barbell Company (California). You can also add resistance for kicking exercises by putting on a man's heavy work shoe.

For the back of the hips and upper thighs, lie prone (face down) and lift one leg as high as you can, backward. Unless you're unusually flexible, you won't get the foot very high off the floor, but keep the leg straight and raise it as high as you can. Try to feel the muscles of the hip and upper thigh tense as you raise the leg. Start with five prone kicks with each leg. After a week, do five with the right leg, five with the left leg, and then repeat five more with each leg. When you repeat an exercise, it's called doing sets, so with the prone kicks you should be doing two sets with each leg, alternately. Try to increase the repetitions to ten per set, staying with two sets for each leg.

STRAIGHT LEG KICKS TO THE SIDE

For the sides of the hips and upper thighs, lie on your side and do the kicks. Raise your leg as far to the side as you can and try to hold your foot in a horizontal position to focus the action on the side of the hip. That is, try not to rotate your leg so the foot points up. If you allow the leg to rotate, the work shifts toward the front instead of working the side of the hip.

Do five kicks to each side at the start and then increase to two sets to each side. Try to increase the repetitions gradually to 15 in each set of this exercise.

SUPINE PRESS ON BENCH

The bench press, as it's called for short, is an excellent exercise for the arms, shoulders, and the pectoral muscles of the chest. It has an effect like doing push-ups, except that you can start with very little resistance and get a better range of mo-

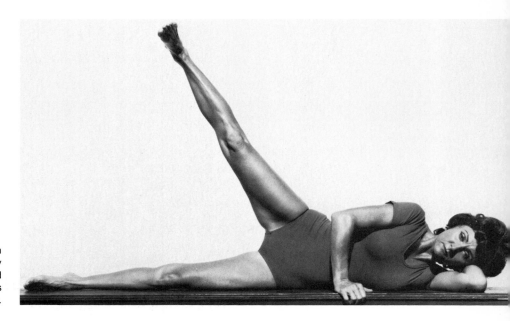

Kicks to the side, as shown, firm the sides of the hips. The intensity of the exercise can be increased by wearing weighted metal sandals or ankle weights.

tion, especially if you use a pair of dumb-bells.

To do the bench press, you lie supine (on your back) on a bench and start with a barbell or a pair of dumbbells held at straight arms directly over your chest, using an overhand grip. If you were using dumbbells, that would mean that the handles would be pointing toward each other, as though they were connected.

Bend your arms with elbows out to the sides and lower the barbell to touch at the mid-chest area, above the breasts, and immediately push it back up to straight arms. Continue for ten repetitions, inhaling as you lower the weight and exhaling as you push it up. With dumbbells, touch the outer edge of the upper chest (near your shoulders) with the inner part of the dumbbells and then push them back up.

Unless you are using very light weights that you can handle easily, you will need someone to hand you the barbell or dumbbells and take the weight away after you have finished the bench presses. There are benches available with uprights where you can place the barbell for convenience in starting bench presses, but even with this apparatus it is advisable to

have someone stand by and "spot" you in case you have trouble completing a press. You should never attempt a bench press you aren't sure you can complete when you're alone.

In the bench press, experiment with very light weights until you find a weight that provides a sensation of muscular effort in the arms, shoulders, and chest, a weight that is fairly difficult to handle for the full ten repetitions. When that weight becomes easy to work with, add five or ten pounds.

Unless you are training for athletic competition in an event like the shot put, or are interested in seeing how much you can lift as a personal challenge, you will find that you will level off with a weight of from 20 to 50 pounds (total weight of bar and plates, or of two dumbbells.) That's plenty for a woman to use for fitness and the muscle tone needed to improve appearance.

THE FLYING EXERCISE FOR TONING PECTORALS AND FIRMING THE BUST

Learned physiologists will insist that it isn't possible to increase bust size. Perhaps they're right in a sense, but it is possible to improve the appearance of the bust by strengthening and toning the pectoral muscles of the chest. These muscles, which stretch from the shoulders to the center of the chest, add fullness or roundness between the breasts and clavicles (collarbones) when properly exercised. This creates an illusion that the breasts are larger even if the actual bust size is unchanged. There is no better single exercise to accomplish this purpose than the bent-arm lateral raise with dumbbells, lying supine (on your back)—called flying because the arm action is like the inverted motion of a bird's wings.

Begin the exercise by lying supine on a bench, holding the dumbbells straight up over your chest with your palms in (toward each other). Bend your arms slightly. Keep your arms in the slightly bent position and lower the dumbbells to the sides as far as you can comfortably stretch. Immediately bring the dumbbells back up and together, as though you were gathering a lot of loosely dispersed things in front of you, or as though you were a bird trying to fly upside down. It is a wide, sweeping motion, not a press; so you must keep elbows bent to minimize strain, but not bent so far that you feel the work in your arms instead of the pectoral muscles of your chest.

Inhale as you lower the weights to the sides and exhale as you bring them back together again. To shift the work to the upper part of the pectorals, which has an uplifting effect, elevate the head end of the bench on a board two inches thick, or on two boards.

Do ten repetitions in the flying motion, using dumbbells just heavy enough to produce a good stretching effect. A pair of three-pounders (the weight of unloaded dumbbell handles if you're using an adjustable set) may be enough to start with but you will probably have to move up to five-pounders in time, and may need to go on to sevens or tens eventually to continue to get good results. After a half-dozen workouts, do two sets of ten.

THE LEG-RAISE, FOR THE LOWER PART OF THE ABDOMEN

The sit-up, described earlier, is an excellent abdominal exerciser, but if you want to activate the lower part of the abdomen more intensively, the leg-raise is one of the best ways to do it. Lie supine (on your

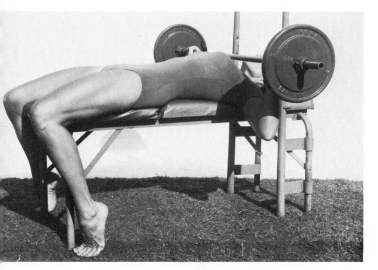
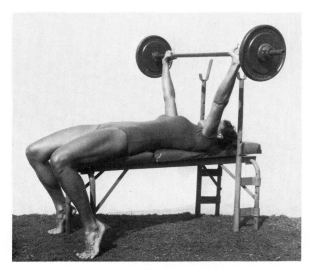

The bench press begins and ends at straight arms. It isn't necessary to use as much weight as Doris Barrilleaux is easily handling in the picture, but enough should be used to give the pectoral (chest) muscles a good workout in eight to ten repetitions.

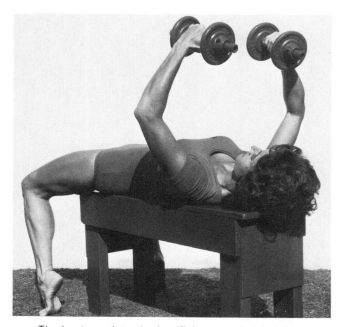 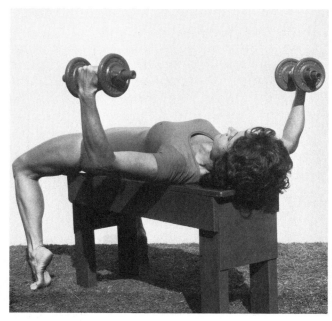

The bent-arm lateral raise (flying exercise) is like the inverted motion of a bird's wings and provides the pectoral muscles full stretch and contraction.

Leg-raising, demonstrated by Linda Carpenter, is an excellent exercise to prevent protrusion of the lower part of the abdomen. It can be made more difficult by attaching weights to the feet.

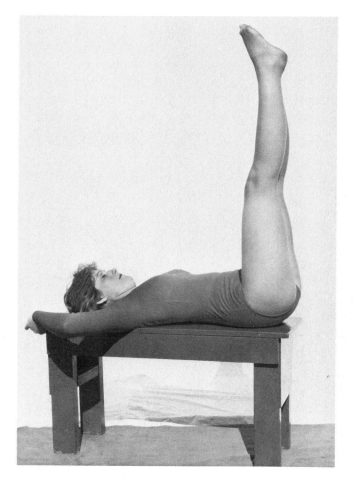

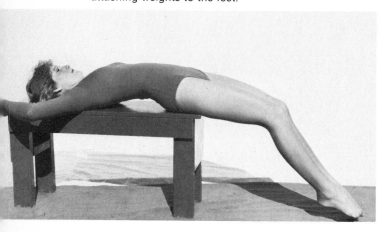

back) on a bench supported only to the hips. Grip the sides of the bench, bend your knees very slightly (and hold the same bend throughout), consciously pull your abdomen in, and raise your legs until they point straight up. Lower them immediately until your feet touch the floor and continue for five to ten repetitions. If you can't do five, repeat sets of two or three to a total of ten. Add repetitions gradually to 20 or 30.

RISE-ON-TOES, FOR SHAPELY CALVES

To improve the shape of the lower legs, stand with your toes and the balls of your feet on a two-inch thick board, so your heels stretch down to reach the floor. Hold a barbell across your shoulders or a dumbbell in each hand, at your sides. (Incidentally, when you're holding a bar-

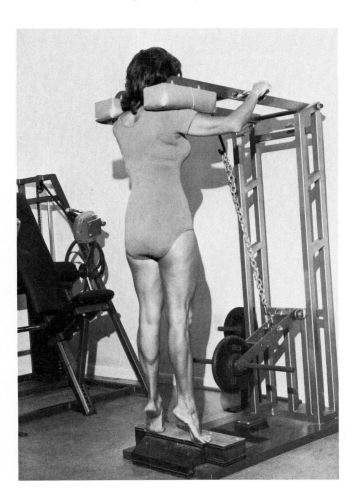

bell across your shoulders for an exercise such as squats or the rise-on-toes, keep it low—below the protruding vertebra at the base of your neck. If it's still uncomfortable, wrap a towel around the center of the bar for padding.)

With the balls of your feet elevated, rise as high as you can on your toes and then lower your heels to touch the floor. Continue alternately rising on toes and touching your heels to the floor ten to 15 repetitions. You may feel some soreness in your calf muscles when you first do the exercise, but after they get used to the work and the stretch, you may need to go on to 20 or 25 repetitions to get a good effect from the exercise. The calf muscles are tough from walking and can take a lot of work. For variety and to fully round out the calves, turn your toes in (heels out) for five to ten reps, toes out (heels together) for five to ten, and point them straight ahead for five to ten.

In addition to the weight-training exercises, anyone interested in general health and fitness should do something that provides sustained exercise for from ten minutes to a half hour, two or three days each week. An intense exercise such as rope-skipping or jogging is effective in from 10 to 15 minutes. Riding a stationary exercise bicycle (with tension turned up) at a steady 15-miles-per-hour pace or faster will have a similar effect. Steady walking or easy outdoor bicycling for 15 minutes to a half hour are other exercises that are good for conditioning your heart and cardiovascular system (and for burning off a few extra calories).

All of the exercises described can be done from one to three sets each, three

To be really effective, the rise-on-toes must be done against resistance. The photo shows a special piece of gym equipment in use, but the exercise can be done with a barbell across the shoulders or while holding dumbbells in the hands.

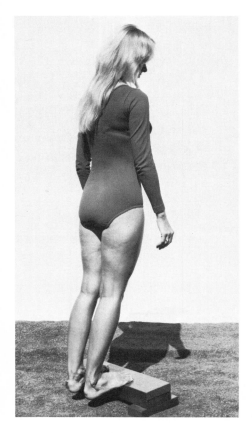
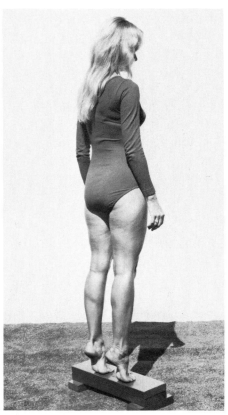

Joyce Weir shows the range of
motion required for best results in
the rise-on-toes exercise. There is
benefit from doing this exercise
without resistance, but even the
minimal added weight of a pair of
dumbbells in the hands makes it
more effective.

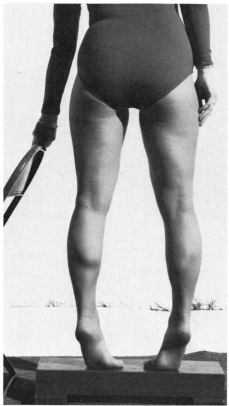
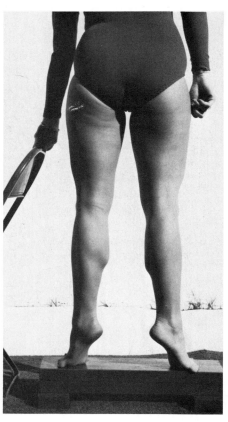

Note the different ways in which
the lower legs are worked when
the toes are pointed in and out.

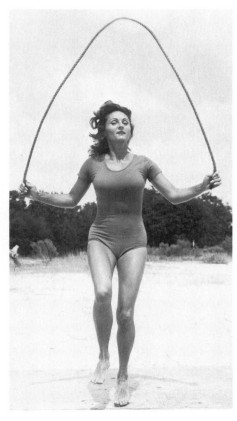

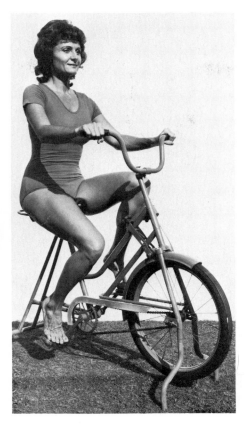

Rope skipping (far left) is a good exercise for the legs, but even better for the heart and lungs. It improves overall cardiorespiratory fitness.

Regular use of a stationary bicycle, 10 to 20 minutes at a time, daily or every other day, helps keep the heart and circulation working efficiently.

days per week. A young woman with a good figure can maintain it with one set of each exercise. Add sets in the exercises that affect the parts of your body that most need improvement. The cardiovascular exercises are included primarily for their benefit to health. If you have a problem with overweight, you need more total exercise, though you probably will need to work into it very gradually. Underweight is another problem. Overweight and underweight will be dealt with in Chapters 3 and 4.

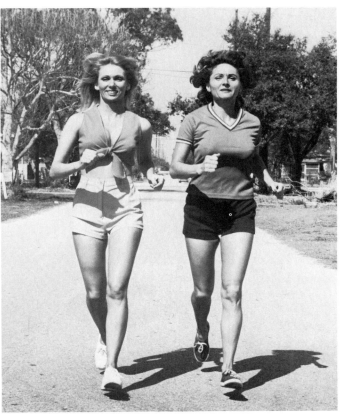

When weather permits, 10 minutes to a half-hour of outdoor jogging provides aerobic conditioning and also uses up a lot of calories.

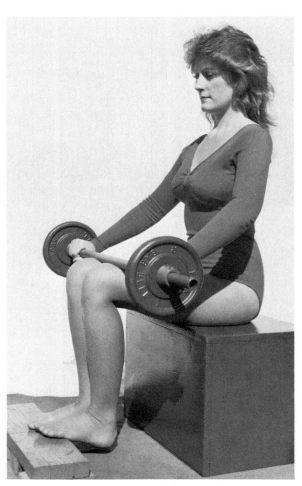 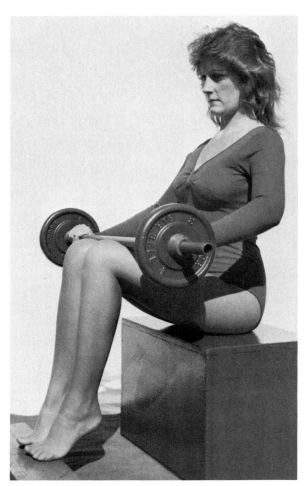

Linda Carpenter demonstrates the rise-on-toes in the seated position, a variation that affects the lower part of the calves.

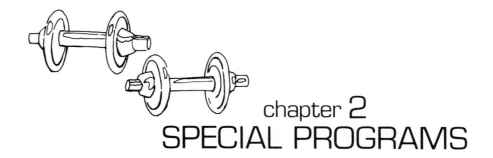

chapter 2
SPECIAL PROGRAMS

A number of special figure problems often experienced by women can be solved or partially solved by applications of weight training. Improved shapeliness of the legs will result from the basic squatting and rise-on-toes exercises, for example, but certain specific areas of the legs may need additional attention.

EXERCISES FOR THE LEGS

The rise-on-toes, seated

The regular rise-on-toes, described in Chapter 1, The Basic Program, works the entire calf area, but it is most effective for the upper part, near the knee. If your lower calf, near the ankle, is underdeveloped or shapeless, you may need to do the rise-on-toes in a seated position. When the knees are bent, the lower portion of the calf (soleus) works harder; when the legs are straight, the upper portion (gastrocnemius) is more strongly involved.

To do the seated rise-on-toes, sit so that you can place the balls of your feet and toes on a fairly thick piece of board. The board should be thick enough to provide a good stretch to the Achilles tendon at the back of your heel. Hold a well-padded barbell across your thighs and perform the rise-on-toes in a seated position as shown in the illustration.

To concentrate on the inner portion of the lower leg, roll your feet toward the outer edges and your little toe as you reach the highest part of the rise. To concentrate on the outer portion, roll your feet so that you are pushing from the base of your big toe at the highest part of the rise.

Do the seated rise-on-toes up to three sets of from 15 to 30 repetitions. Try three foot positions: toes in, toes out, and toes pointed straight ahead.

If your lower calf is very underdeveloped, do all your rise-on-toes movements seated. If the disproportion is only slight, include the regular standing rise-on-toes as well.

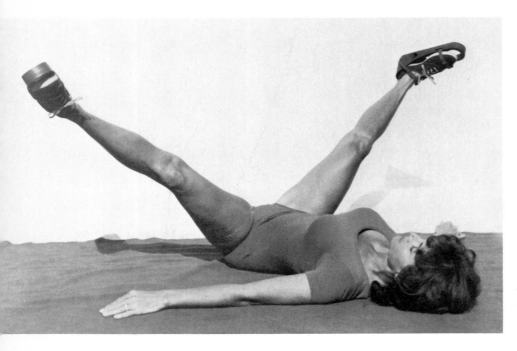

To fill in hollows along the inner thigh, a sideways scissors motion with weights on the feet is called for.

Exercise for the inner thigh

Many women are plagued by flabbiness or lack of development along the inside of the thighs. If this problem is not solved by doing squats with weights, it may be necessary to practice a direct exercise for the adductors—the muscles that draw the thighs together.

Do the exercise lying supine (on your back). Attach weights to your feet or ankles. Brace your hands alongside your hips for balance and point your legs straight up, feet together. Then spread your legs as far to the sides as they will go and bring them back together. Repeat ten times.

To provide resistance for the leg-spread exercise, you can use a pair of metal sandals (called "iron boots" or "health shoes") or ankle weights. The sandals are better, because they are designed to hold a dumbbell bar and thus the weight can be increased if you feel that you need added resistance. Both ankle weights and metal sandals are available at sporting goods stores, or you can order from such sources as the York Barbell Company, York, Pennsylvania; the Weider Barbell Company, Woodland Hills, California; the Iron Man Barbell Company, Alliance, Nebraska; the Lurie Barbell Company, Brooklyn, New York; or other exercise equipment suppliers that sell by mail order.

Proceed cautiously with stretching movements such as the leg spread, especially the first few times you do the exercise, or you'll wind up with very sore muscles. As you get used to it, however, you can try for more stretch, add sets to a total of three, and increase the resistance from five pounds to ten or more.

Exercise for the back of the thigh

Any exercise in which you bend forward and then straighten again, such as a dead-weight lift, good-morning exercise, or hyperextension, has some effect on the backs of your thighs. To work the area specifically and directly, however, you have to use a special leg-curling apparatus available in health clubs or perform a leg-curling motion with metal sandals or ankle weights.

Attach a weight to one foot or ankle and stand with the other foot raised off the floor, on a stair step, thick block of wood, or a sturdy box or stool. Hold onto something to help maintain balance and bend the leg with the weight attached so that you raise the weighted foot up behind you as far as possible. Lower and repeat ten times; then switch the weight to the other foot and exercise the other leg.

As you do the leg curls, try to keep your thigh hanging straight down and to pull the weighted foot up behind you as far as the knee will bend. Extend the leg fully (to point straight down) after each curl. This exercise tones the entire back of the thigh from your hip to the back of your knee.

Leg extensions for the frontal thigh

An excellent exercise for the front part of the thigh is also done with weighted sandals. You sit on a sturdy table, supported to the knees and with lower legs hanging down, weights attached to your feet. In this position, simply extend your legs fully until your knees are locked. Repeat ten times, up to three sets. This exercise tones the entire front of the thigh and also strengthens the muscles that help stabilize the knee joint. The exercise helps prevent knee injury and also is useful for rehabilitation after a knee has been injured.

EXERCISE FOR IMPROVED BUST SHAPE
Incline bench presses and raises

The regular bench press and flying exercises (bent-arm lateral raise) are unexcelled movements to strengthen and tone the pectoral muscles that lift and improve the shape of the bust. To provide additional work for this area, however, the same exercises should be done on an incline. Special benches are available for these exercises in health clubs, but you can do them at home by placing a thick

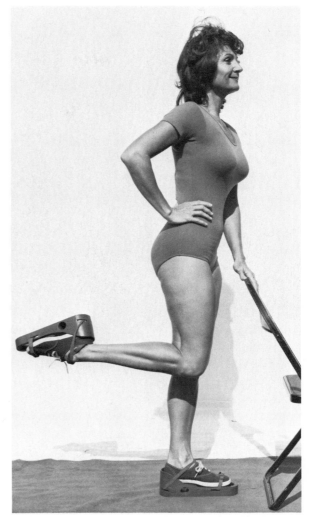

Shapeliness of the back of the thigh can be improved by a leg curling motion with weight on the foot.

block of wood under the head end of a regular flat bench, or you can brace a sturdy board against a wall, providing it is braced securely at the bottom.

Incline bench presses can be done with a barbell or two dumbbells, but dumbbells have two advantages: (1) They're easier to swing into position to start pressing, and (2) they can be lowered to the sides of your shoulders and thus provide more stretch for the shoulder muscles and the upper part of the pectoral muscles that you are trying to activate.

Do the exercise this way: Pick up two

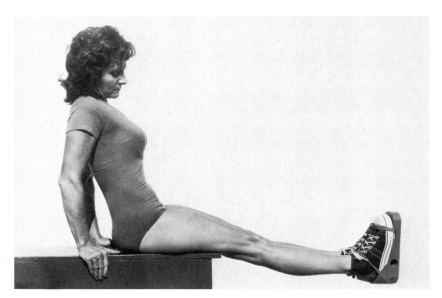

The fronts of the thighs are worked strongly, and the muscles stabilizing the knees are strengthened by leg extensions with resistance.

dumbbells—about five pounds each, to start—and brace your feet at the bottom of the inclined bench or board, your legs and hips against the board, but with your torso upright. Lean forward slightly and then lean back, swinging the dumbbells to your shoulders as your back reaches the support. Turn the dumbbells so that the inside ends point approximately at your ears. Inhale and push the dumbbells smoothly upward and inward so that the inner ends touch or almost touch as your arms straighten, pointing straight up. Exhale as your arms straighten. As soon as your arms are straight, lower the dumbbells, inhaling, to touch the outer edge of your shoulders and immediately press them again. Continue for eight to ten repetitions. If you can't complete eight, you're trying to use too much weight. As you become accustomed to the exercise, add sets to a total of three sets of ten repetitions. When the exercise becomes too easy, add weight, although few women will want to proceed to any heavier weights than ten- to 15-pound dumbbells.

You can also use a barbell for incline presses, starting the press from the upper chest near the collarbones. Note that although you are pushing the weight straight up, it is actually traveling at an angle, the same angle as the incline of the bench. The more upright the bench, the more your shoulders work and the more the effort is focused on the uppermost part of the pectoral muscles.

To work the upper part of the pectorals with the flying exercise, you perform the exercise the same way as is described in Chapter 1, The Basic Program, except that the angle of the bench shifts the focus of the activity toward the upper portion of the pectoral muscles.

FIRMING AND FLATTENING THE UPPER BACK

As the years go by, most women have a tendency to develop an unsightly bulge at the base of the neck. This bulge is called "dowager's hump." To minimize the hump, it is important to maintain good muscle tone in the muscles of the upper back, especially the trapezius muscles running from the neck to the shoulders, the latissimus muscles that draw the arms down and back, and the muscles at the center of the upper back that draw the shoulders back and the shoulder blades together.

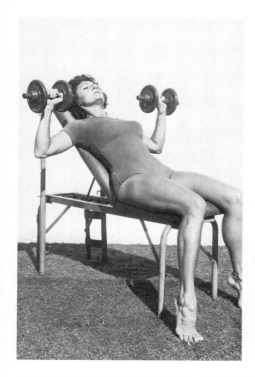
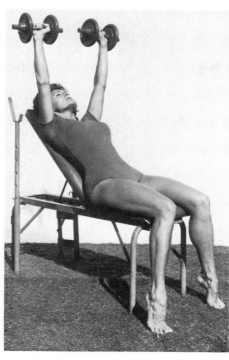

Pressing weights on a steep incline affects the upper part of the chest muscles, improving the shape of the bust.

The upper pectorals are toned by the flying exercise on an incline, creating a high chested look.

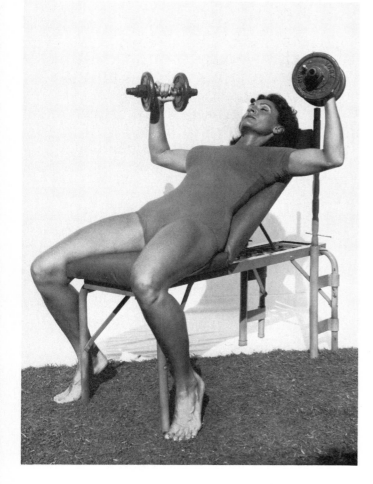

Two exercises that can be practiced with a barbell or two dumbbells at home are particularly good for maintaining muscle tone in the upper back area. One is the regular rowing motion, in which you bend forward from the hips until your back is horizontal, bending your knees slightly to relieve strain on your low back and the backs of your legs. Hold a light barbell (about 20 pounds) with an overhand grip, hands spaced slightly wider than shoulder width (or hold a pair of dumbbells, about ten pounds each, hanging straight down) with the weight hanging at straight arms below your shoulders. Pull the weight(s) up and toward your abdomen so that the barbell touches at the bottom of your chest (dumbbells are pulled up with the same motion, slightly higher, to the sides of the bottom of your rib cage). Lower the weight(s) and continue for a total of at least eight repetitions. As you become

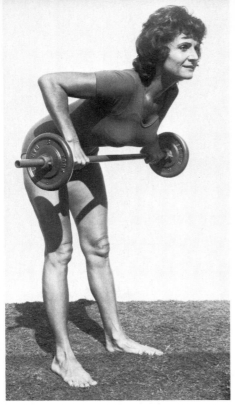

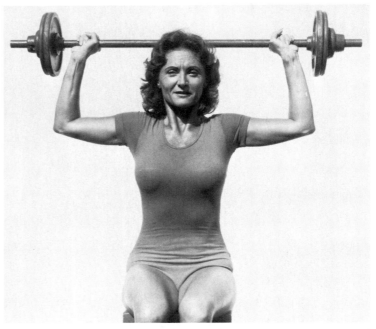

Practice of a rowing motion while leaning forward strengthens upper back muscles.

Pressing a barbell from low behind the neck helps flatten the upper back and tones muscles that counteract "dowager's hump."

accustomed to the exercise, increase the repetitions to ten and add sets to three.

The second exercise that can be done easily at home is the press behind neck with barbell, or a variation with dumbbells that we'll describe later. With a barbell, starting with a total weight of 15 to 25 pounds, clean (lift) the bar to your chest, using an overhand grip with hands spaced about four to six inches wider than shoulder width. Push (press) the barbell overhead. Then lower it behind your neck to touch low on the backs of your shoulders and push it back up to straight arms. Continue to press the weight up and down behind your neck a total of 10 repetitions (each time it reaches straight arms overhead counts as one press behind neck). Make an effort to pull your shoulders back as you lower the weight to touch well down on your upper back, below the base of your neck.

To do the exercise with dumbbells, you have to concentrate a bit more on performance. Hold two dumbbells at your shoulders and turn them so the handles point straight out from your ears. Press them overhead. Lower them, simultaneously drawing your shoulders back so that the dumbbells touch the outer edge of the backs of your shoulders at the lowest point. Push them back overhead and continue for a total of ten repetitions. Whether you're pressing a barbell or dumbbells, start with a weight you can handle for at least eight repetitions, add repetitions to ten, and add sets to three.

If you have access to a gym or health club, you may want to substitute lat pulls, an exercise in which you pull a bar (usually curved) from full stretch overhead to a point low behind your neck. A lat machine provides a pulley weight that works the muscles in much the same way as chinning the bar, except that you can use much less than your own weight to start. This exercise can be substituted for rowing and should also be done three sets of ten repetitions.

If you find that the press and either

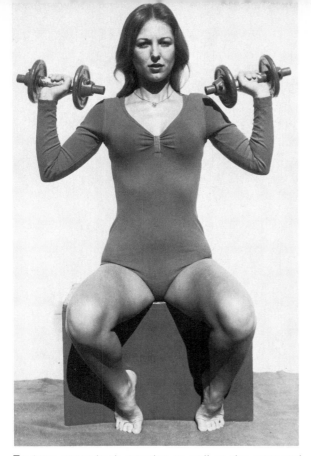

To tone upper back muscles as well as the arms and shoulders, the dumbbells should be pulled well back throughout the pressing exercise. Anne Leto shows the correct starting position.

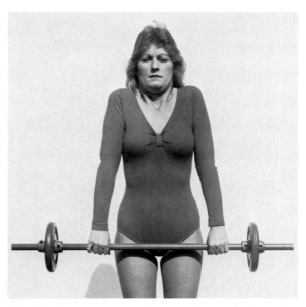

The simplest way to tone the muscles running from the neck to the shoulders is to hold a barbell or two dumbbells and shrug as high as possible, as though to touch shoulders to ears.

rowing or lat pull exercises do not provide enough exercise for the upper back region, you can also do a shrugging movement. In this exercise, you stand and hold two dumbbells hanging at your sides or a barbell hanging with your arms straight and the bar across your thighs. Allowing your arms to hang straight throughout, simply shrug your shoulders as high as possible, attempting to touch your ears. Continue for a total of ten shrugs, three sets. Also try shrugging your shoulders in a rotating motion, up to the front and down to the back, then reverse the rotation.

For variety, try the upright rowing motion. In this, you hold a barbell across your thighs with a narrow overhand grip (hands about six to 12 inches apart) and pull the bar up to your throat, keeping your elbows up throughout. This exercise should also be done three sets of ten.

KNEE-UPS FOR THE LOWER ABDOMEN

If you find that regular sit-ups and leg-raises don't provide enough exercise to flatten a bulge in the lower abdomen, try knee-ups. These can be done on an inclined exercise board or—with greater difficulty—while hanging from a chinning bar.

Performance is simple. Hold the strap or T-bar at the elevated end of an exercise bench (or a chinning bar) and start from a completely stretched-out position, legs extended. Then inhale, exhale, and draw up both knees as far as possible. Lower and repeat five to ten times. Make a real effort to pull your knees all the way up to your chest. This is a difficult exercise and

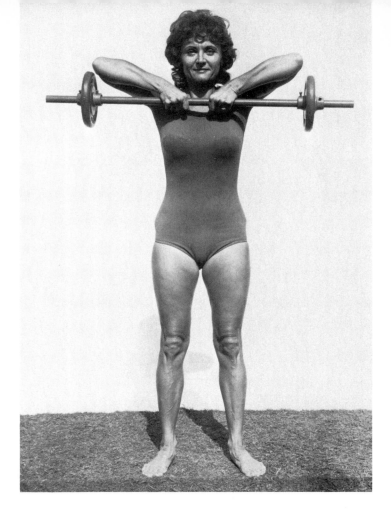

A particularly effective exercise for the shoulders and upper back muscles (trapezius) is the upright rowing motion.

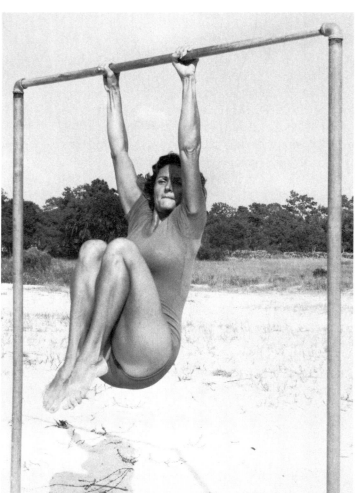

Doris Barrilleaux demonstrates the most advanced way to do the knee-up exercise. This can be done flat on the floor and on increasingly steep inclined boards for progressive effects.

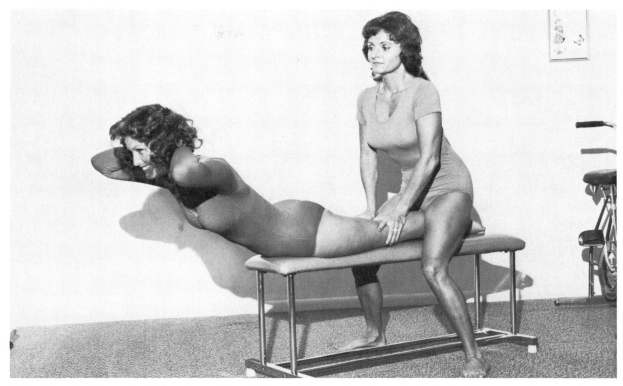

Cindy Henning shows the high arch position of the back hyperextension, with Doris Barrilleaux serving as anchorperson.

contracts the abdominal muscles more thoroughly than any other single movement. So you may find you can't do very many of these the first time you try the exercise, even if you've progressed to where you can do 20 or more sit-ups or leg-raises. Persist, however, even if you can only do two or three at a time before stopping to rest. Continue in sets until you have completed a dozen (for example: three, three, three, two, one) and keep trying to add repetitions every time you exercise. It will be most unusual if you haven't flattened your lower tummy noticeably by the time you can do three sets of ten.

HYPEREXTENSIONS FOR THE LOW BACK

Some people have very vulnerable low backs, suffering frequent lumbosacral sprains and strains. This is the injury that occurs as a sudden "catch" near the center or a bit off center just above the buttocks. Sometimes the immediate injury isn't noticed, but progressively increasing pain and stiffness develops in the area. If you have this tendency but there is no serious orthopedic or neurologic problem, you can probably improve the condition by doing a simple exercise called the hyperextension. (Your doctor can tell you if you have an injury, such as a herniated disc, that would prevent you from such exercising.)

The back hyperextension is done in the prone (face down) position. There are several pieces of apparatus for doing hyperextensions in gyms and health clubs, but you can improvise at home and do them across a hassock, the edge of a bed, or at the top of stairs. You should place a pad under your pelvic area, and you will need someone to hold down your feet as you support yourself on your pelvis and upper thighs (and legs, if you're lying on a bench, across a bed, or at the top of stairs).

Your upper torso should extend well out from the support, so that you can let your body hang down and then arch upward. That's all the exercise consists of: bending forward then arching up while in the prone position.

If you have the typical "touchy" low back, you may not be able to do the forward bending movements described in Chapter 1, The Basic Program, and you probably won't be able to do straight-leg raises or sit-ups with legs straight, either. But you should be able to do hyperextensions. This is because your weight is hanging down from your spine in the prone position, not placing any vertical mechanical stress on the supporting structures of the low back. In this position, the raising and lowering motion directly works the muscles that run along the spine and other allied muscles of the area. The exercise strengthens the weak area specifically, building muscular support.

Incidentally, if you find that arching up high causes discomfort, just raise to the point where your head is as high as or slightly higher than your hips.

The hyperextension exercise should be done in three sets of eight to ten repetitions and should be done in conjunction with bent-knee sit-ups. (Do the sit-ups carefully, too; even though your knees are bent, be sure to roll up into the sitting position, rather than levering up from the hips with a stiff back.)

You should try to hold weight behind your head in the hyperextension and, ideally, your goal is to be able to hyperextend ten repetitions with three times as much weight behind your head as you can sit up with. For example, if you do sit-ups without weight, you should strive to do hyperextensions with a two-and-one-half- to three-pound weight behind your head.

If you can sit up with five pounds for ten reps, you should try to work up to do ten hyperextensions with a 15-pound weight behind your head.

If you have been a person with chronic low back problems not due to a serious medical condition, you will very likely find that your trouble has cleared up by the time you can do bent-knee sit-ups with two-and-one-half to three pounds behind your head and hyperextensions with ten pounds. To prevent a recurrence of the trouble, try to reach a level of strength in which you can do the sit-ups with five to ten pounds and the hyperextensions with 15 to 30 pounds.

FOR THE HIPS AND SIDES

The twisting exercise, and the kicks to the side and to the rear in the prone position are excellent exercises for the hips and sides (described in Chapter 1, The Basic Program). But when more work is needed for these areas, there are several additional movements that should be helpful.

One is done on all fours or, rather, kneeling on one knee and both hands. In an all-fours position, pick up one knee and draw the knee as far forward toward your chin as you can, lowering your head to meet it. Then extend the same leg backward and up as far and high as you can reach. Repeat five times—knee to chest, then extend the leg back and up—and then do five with the other leg. Strive to extend the leg up and back so that you feel tension in the hip area. Repeat the exercise in sets, five with the right leg, five with the left; five more with the right, five more with the left. When it becomes easy to do three sets of five with each leg, begin to increase the repetitions until you can do at least three sets of ten with each leg.

Another good exercise for the sides is to sit on the floor with legs outstretched. Hold your arms out to the sides and do

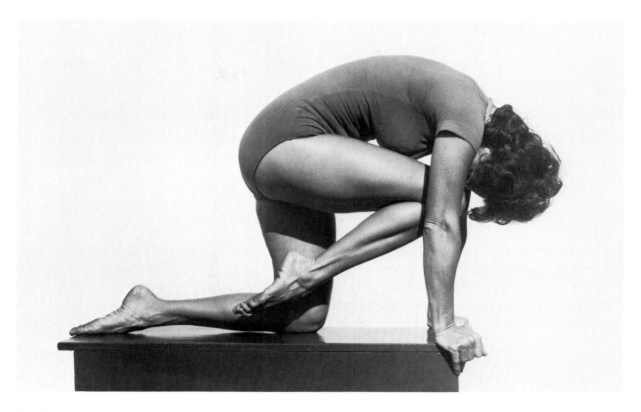

Kneeling back kicks, as shown, work waist, hips, and lower back. The exercise is effective without weights, but can be made tougher by wearing a metal sandal or an ankle weight.

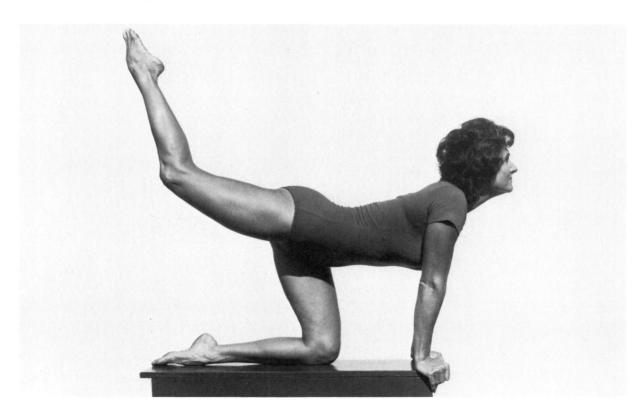

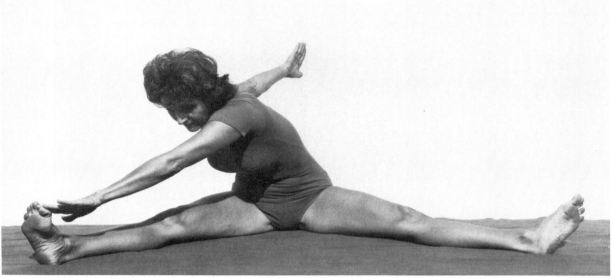

Alternate twisting toe-touching, seated: a fine waist-tightening free-hand exercise.

an alternate twisting toe-touch, reaching for your left foot with your right arm and vice versa. Work up from ten to 50 repetitions.

In the same position, seated with legs outstretched, reach to touch your toes alternately with *both* hands, deliberately stretching your sides and the upper part of your hips. Work up from ten to 20 repetitions.

A variation on the side kicks given in the basic program should also be helpful. In this one, you lie on your side and perform straight leg kicks as high to the side as possible, but angle the kicks to the front slightly and to the rear slightly, alternately, instead of kicking directly to the side. Do ten to each side and repeat up to three sets if the sides of your hips need trimming and shaping.

Two more good movements are the alternate toe touch, bending forward from the hips, and cross-leg swings while lying supine. The cross-leg swings are done while lying with arms outstretched to the sides. In that position, swing your right leg over as far as possible, as though to touch your left hand, and then swing your left leg over toward your right hand.

Work up from ten to 20 repetitions in both exercises.

HIP AND THIGH TONER

Most of the waist, hip, and thigh toning exercises can be done freehand (without added resistance, that is). A good thigh toner that can be done without weights or while holding a light barbell (the barbell handle is plenty of resistance, especially at the start) is the lunge. You start in a standing position and take a long step forward with one leg, bending the knee to approximately a right angle, stretching the other leg. Step forward with the back leg, rising, and then repeat the lunge forward with the other leg. Turn and repeat two lunges, with alternate legs. Again, turn and repeat until you have completed five lunges with each leg. Increase the repetitions until you can do ten with each leg.

Lunges can be repeated in sets to three, and you can increase the effectiveness of the exercise by adding weight to the barbell (or by holding a pair of dumbbells at your sides) as three sets of ten with each leg becomes easy.

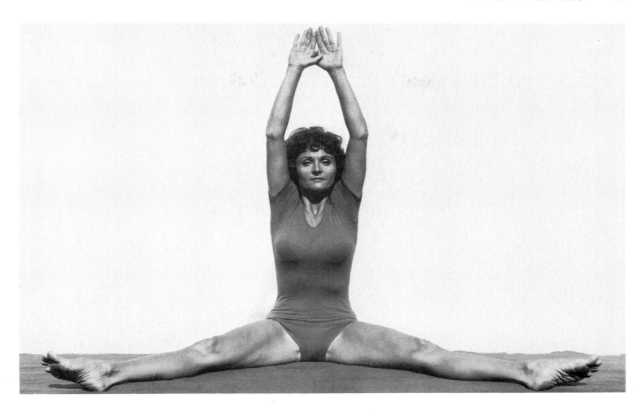

An advanced exercise for the sides of the waist and the hips is this stretching two-hands toe-touch, seated.

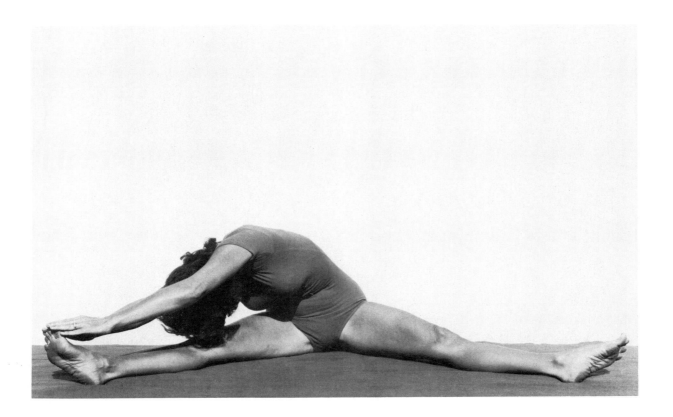

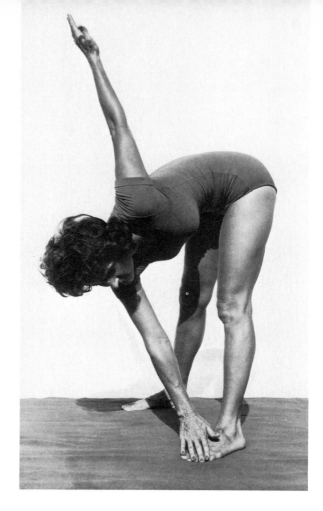

The alternate toe-touch, standing, is a good exercise for the waist, upper hips, and low back.

A vigorous, result-producing leg and hip exercise is the lunge, practiced with alternate legs. Lunges can be made more difficult—and more effective—by holding dumbbells or a light barbell (across the shoulders).

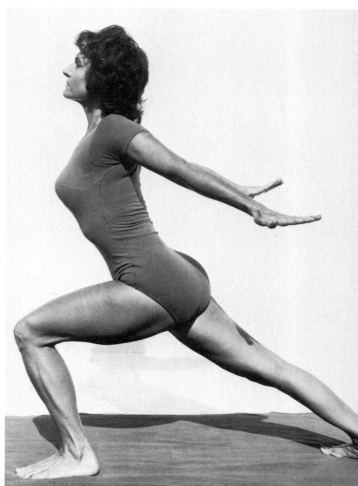

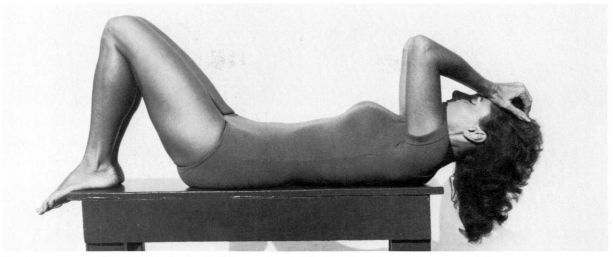

Hand pressure, as shown, tones the front of the neck and chin. The head is moved up against the pressure.

EXERCISES FOR THE FACE AND NECK

The face and neck are affected to some extent by any arm and shoulder exercise in which there is effort, but a more youthful appearance can be maintained by deliberately performing some simple exercises for them. For the front of the neck and chin, lie supine (on your back), place your hands against your forehead, and raise your head to bring your chin to your chest, resisting with your hands. Repeat 20 times. If you have double-chin problems, do the exercise several times a day.

Another good one is to simply rotate your head around in a full range of motion, moving your jaw in the same direction that your head is going. Still another is to fold a light towel into a strip, place it in your mouth, and pull down on both ends while tensing your jaw against the pull and moving your head up and down, and side to side.

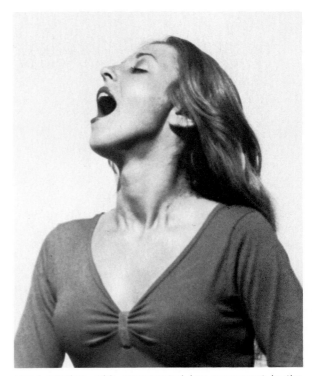

Head rotation, with exaggerated jaw movement in the direction of the rotation, tones face, neck, and chin.

IMPORTANCE OF MENTAL ATTITUDE

As you tackle special figure problems, remember that your mental attitude is important. You have to form a mental picture of the body part that you want to improve, concentrating on involving it strongly in the exercise. If you want to tighten and firm your abdomen, you have to picture it firm and taut, and you have to force the abdominal muscles to pull in as you draw your legs up or sit up.

The same is true with the other exercises. You've got to think of squared

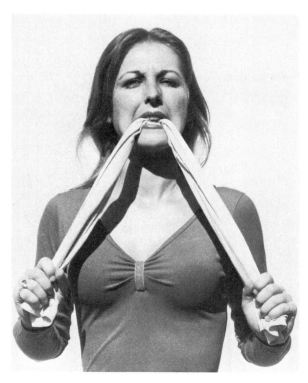

Anne Leto is using a folded towel to apply resistance as she raises and lowers her head and jaw.

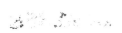

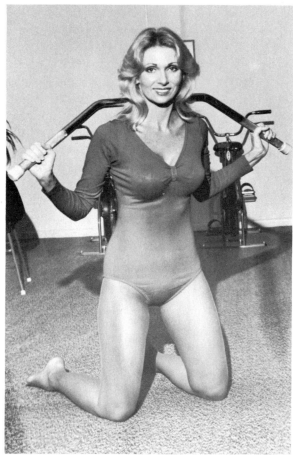

Well-equipped gyms provide convenient equipment, such as the lat machine Joyce Weir is pulling down in one of the most effective upper back exercises.

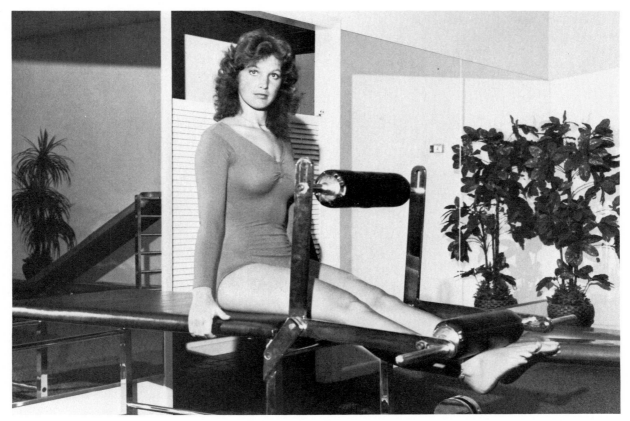

Cindy Henning demonstrates the leg extension, an excellent thigh firmer, on a machine at Hector's and Elisa's Health Studio in Tampa, Florida.

shoulders and a flattened back as you lower the weight before pressing. You've got to concentrate on the stretch and return pull as you work leg adductor muscles against the resistance of weighted health sandals.

If you will learn to get the correct feel of working the proper body part thoroughly, you will get much more out of exercising than if you simply go through the motions—though going through the motions is better than not exercising at all!

USING SPECIAL EQUIPMENT

If you can join a gym or health club where special gym equipment is available, it will make your workouts a lot easier.

You can use the lat machine, for example, for exercises that flatten and tone your upper back. You can do leg curls and extensions on special apparatus that is much more convenient than using weights on your feet or ankles. Many gyms have special bust-developing exercisers that enable you to perform the flying exercise by placing your elbows against padded resistance arms.

The exercises described in this book can be done at home with little special equipment. In fact, you could improvise most of it, though commercially manufactured weights and benches are much more convenient. But many of the exercises can be done even more conveniently with special gym equipment. Exercise at a gym can be fun, since you will find people with

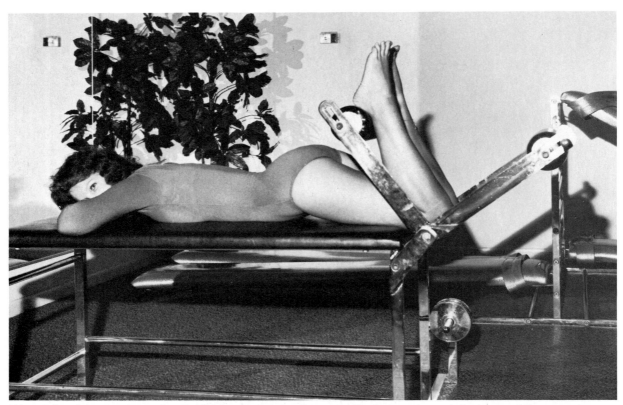

(Above) Special apparatus makes the thigh curl exercise the most effective way to work the backs of the upper legs.

(Below) The flying exercise can be done conveniently on special apparatus designed for toning the bust area.

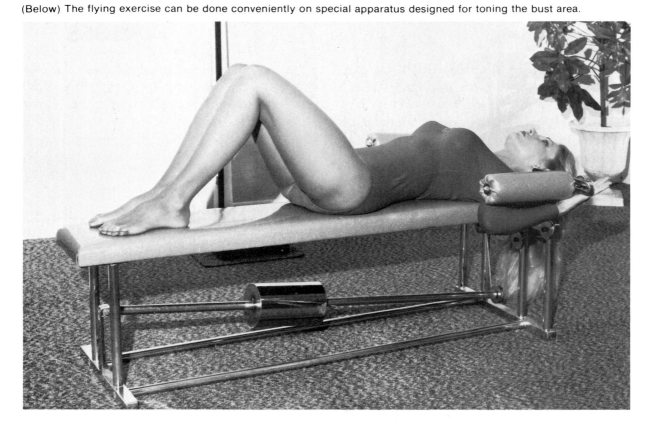

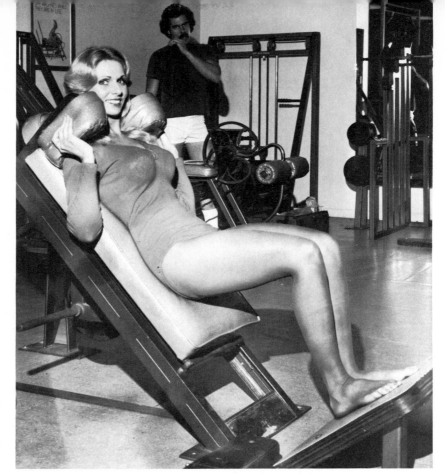

Even squats can be comfortable on a padded, sliding leg exercise machine such as this one at Hector's gym in Tampa.

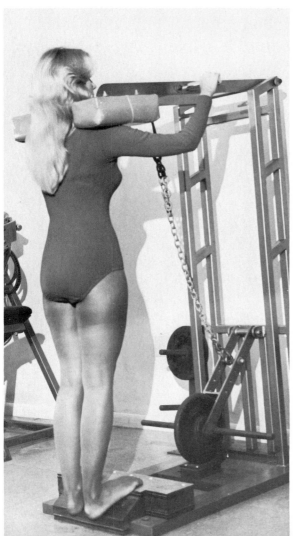

Special calf exercise apparatus makes it possible to work the lower leg muscles vigorously without any difficulty in maintaining balance.

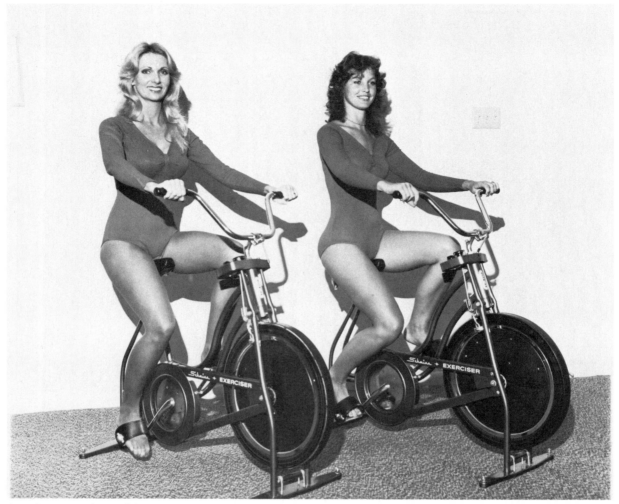

An advantage of exercising at a health club is the fun of working out with other positive thinkers. The pedalers are Joyce Weir (left) and Cindy Henning.

similar interests attempting to overcome similar problems. If the gym is a good one, you'll also have the advantage of instruction though many of the highly commercialized health clubs and spas have "instructors" chosen more for inherent attractiveness and sales ability than for their knowledge of exercise.

Be careful about joining a health club or spa, especially if you get a high-pressure sales pitch, are urged to join "right now," without thinking it over, and if there is a contract to sign. Evaluate the deal that is offered carefully. If you are signing a contract, is it really reasonable over the long run? (Many gyms count on people not using the memberships they pay for; few rates are bargains unless you really use the facilities.) Can the contract be cancelled if you should become ill or move away? Is the gym available to you when you want to use it? (Many gyms have alternate men's and women's hours, or days, which can be inconvenient).

But if you do find that a gym or health club offers facilities that will provide you with the exercise you need, plus instruction and compatible training partners—

and if you can afford it—by all means join and make good use of it. There's nothing like forming a habit pattern of going to a health club for a workout regularly, three days a week or more often, to keep you exercising healthfully.

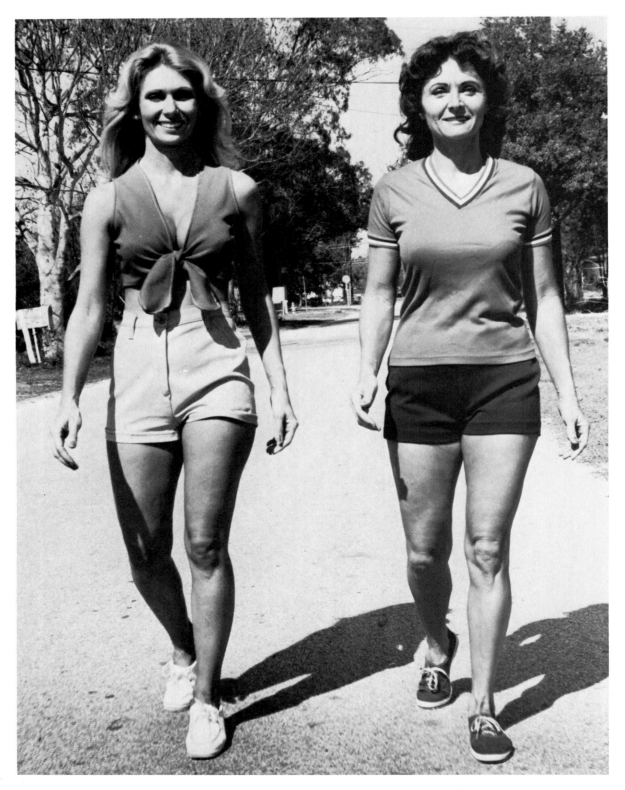

Continuous walking at a brisk pace, for at least a half hour a day (this time can be divided into sessions) is one of the best ways to work off excess weight. Joyce Weir is on the left and Doris Barrilleaux on the right.

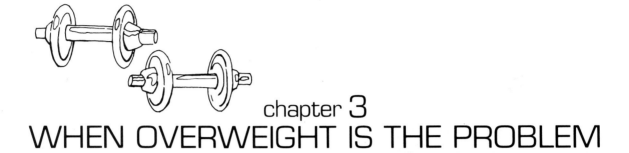

chapter 3
WHEN OVERWEIGHT IS THE PROBLEM

Many women think they're overweight when their real problem is flabbiness and lack of muscle tone. But many are truly overweight . . . and usually out of shape, with poor muscle tone as well. When these problems coexist, it's a lot tougher to get in shape than when there is no problem other than flabbiness. With real overweight, exercise should be started easily and its intensity should be increased very gradually. Speedier results can be achieved by combining dieting with exercise, but there is scientific evidence that you can reduce without dieting if you are willing to greatly increase your activity.

Reducing by exercising is much more satisfactory than reducing by dieting. Dieting is certainly unpleasant for someone who likes to eat, and it also tends to leave your face and body sagging with stretched skin hanging unsupported by toned muscles. When you lose weight while exercising, the underlying muscles become firm and minimize the sag. In fact, you can actually reduce your waist measurement by strengthening your abdominal muscles without losing any weight at all. To remove fat, however, you have to burn up more calories with exercise than you take in by eating and drinking.

To burn calories, you can do the same exercises that are described in the basic program. This will burn calories rather slowly, however, and will call for a lot of dietary discipline in addition to the exercise. To burn the excess calories more quickly, you should follow a very simple program: *Walk briskly at least one-half hour a day.*

You might think that a half-hour of walking a day would not have much effect, but the recommendation is based on a study conducted by Grant Gwinup, M.D., of the Division of Endocrinology and Metabolism, University of California (Irvine). Dr. Gwinup found that when women who were ten to 60 percent overweight would walk at least 30 minutes a day, they would gradually lose weight—from ten to 38 pounds in a year. The average weight loss was 22 pounds, and the women who walked more than a half-hour a day lost the most weight.

Incidentally, Dr. Gwinup's subjects did not do all their walking at one time. In other words, someone walking a half-hour a day might do it ten minutes at a time, three different times a day; or 15 minutes at a time, twice a day. No attempt was made, in Dr. Gwinup's study (reported in the *Archives of Internal Medicine*, Volume 135, May 1975), to restrict diet or count calories. Most of the women thought they actually increased their food intake and Dr. Gwinup believed that this was probably true. He noted that walking produces an energy expenditure of about 300 calories an hour; since body fat contains approximately 3,500 calories per pound, he calculated that those who walked for two hours a day would have lost about 1.25 pounds per week instead of the half-pound or less that they did lose. A half-pound loss per week, of course, adds up to 25 pounds a year, and it must be good news to those with hearty appetites that this much could be lost without dieting.

On the other hand, a little dietary discipline—just halving the amount of bread, pastry, and desserts eaten, for example—would speed the rate of fat loss. Remember that fat in the diet contains about nine calories per gram and alcohol contains seven per gram. By contrast, there are only approximately four calories per gram in protein and carbohydrates. Therefore, you can see that cutting down on alcoholic beverages and fatty meats can have as important an effect on dieting as can cutting down or eliminating desserts. Try eliminating major amounts of visible fat in your diet. Cut away excess fat from meat, and include more fish and poultry. Avoid fried foods and the use of fat in food preparation.

If you are greatly overweight, you will have to begin exercising very gradually, and it would be an excellent idea to check with your doctor first to be sure you have no medical problems that would prevent or limit your undertaking an exercise program. Once you do decide to begin, however, proceed with caution. Start by walking only five minutes at a time. Wear comfortable clothing, especially the shoes. If, after a couple of days, you find that you are not experiencing any unusual discomfort—such as blisters or muscular soreness in the lower legs—increase to two five-minute sessions at widely separated intervals. Say, a five-minute walk in the morning and another in the afternoon. When two five-minute walks become easy, add a third, or increase one of the walks to ten minutes. After two weeks of walking a total of 15 minutes a day, take two ten-minute walks every day of the third week. Then move up to three ten-minute walks or two 15-minute walks. You will then be at the minimum amount of walking it should take for you to lose about a half-pound of fat a week. If you find walking reasonably easy, you might want to add a few minutes to each walking session. Remember, all who walked a half-hour a day lost weight, but those who walked more than a half-hour lost more!

In addition to the walking, ease into some of the weight training exercises. Do sit-ups, without weight at first. If you are more than slightly overweight, you will probably have to start by reaching forward with your arms to help you sit up. Otherwise, do the exercise as described in the basic routine. Lie supine. Tuck your feet under something or have them held down. Bend your knees. Take a breath and then exhale, reaching toward your

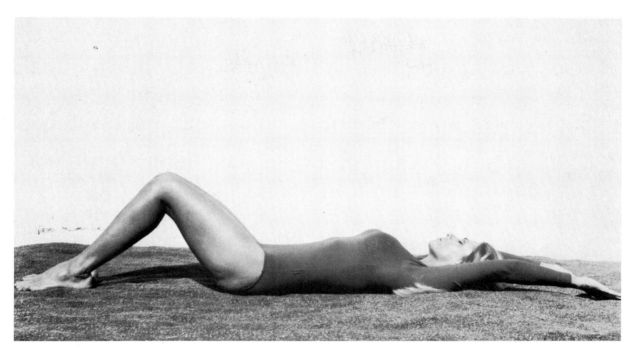

Helping the motion by reaching forward is the easiest way to begin sit-ups. It's easier still when the feet are held down.

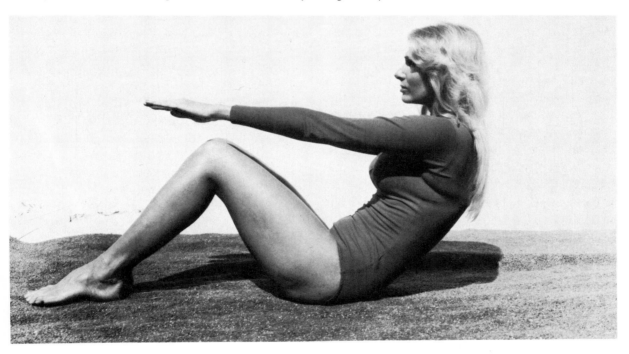

feet, and sit up. Return to the supine position, inhaling. Try to do five to ten sit-ups, even if you have to rest briefly after each one. Keep trying to add sit-ups until you can do 25 without stopping to rest.

After you can do 25 consecutive sit-ups reaching, do them with your arms folded across your chest. This will make them more difficult and you may have to drop back to ten or 15, but persist and work up gradually to 25 with your arms folded. Then do a set of 25, rest awhile and do 15 to 25 more. When you can do two sets of 25, do the sit-ups with your hands clasped behind your neck.

When you can do 20 or more sit-ups with hands clasped behind your neck, you are beginning to develop pretty good abdominal muscle tone and you should be able to see the results, especially when these abdominal exercises are being done in conjunction with a walking program. Do both of these exercises—walking and sit-ups—every day. Walk briskly, consciously keeping your abdomen pulled in. And consciously pull your abdomen in, after exhaling, at the start of *each* sit-up.

After a month of regular walking and abdominal exercise, you should be ready for some more general muscle-toning exercises. These are to be added to your program on alternate days, three days a week, but you should keep up the walking and sit-ups daily.

MUSCLE-TONING IN THE WEIGHT-LOSS PROGRAM

As you lose weight by expending more calories than you are taking in, muscle-toning for every part of your body will greatly improve your appearance. The walking and sit-ups will help tone your legs and abdomen, but you should also do exercises for your arms, chest, back, and shoulders, and additional exercises for your legs.

To start with muscle-toning, try just two exercises three days a week—Monday, Wednesday, and Friday; or Tuesday, Thursday, and Saturday. Remember, you're supposed to be walking and doing sit-ups *every* day. The two exercises are partial knee bends and pull-overs.

Begin the knee bends with no added weight resistance. Stand in front of a chair, feet a comfortable distance apart and hands on hips. Take a breath high in your chest, pull your abdomen in, and bend your knees until your rear touches the chair lightly. Rise immediately. Exhale. Repeat five to ten times. Maintain a very erect position while doing knee bends to the extent of holding your back in an exaggerated arched position. Make the bends a smoothly controlled effort. Keep your feet flat on the floor.

If you find you can do the knee bends ten repetitions with ease, hold dumbbells in your hands or a light barbell across your shoulders. Use enough weight so that it feels fairly difficult to complete six to eight knee bends at first, add one or two each time you exercise, and increase the weight whenever it becomes easy to complete ten repetitions. Obviously, you won't want to keep increasing the weight indefinitely unless you are trying to build strength for a competitive sport. You may find that a maintenance weight of 30 to 50 pounds is as far as you want to go.

In addition to knee bends (squats), do pullovers. In this exercise, you lie supine and hold a light weight (an unloaded barbell handle, one dumbbell of about five to ten pounds, or two small dumbbells) straight up over your chest. Begin to inhale and simultaneously lower the weight (arms straight or very slightly bent) behind your head until it touches the floor. If you do the exercise lying on a bench, lower the weight as far as is comfortable. (Some people find it hurts their

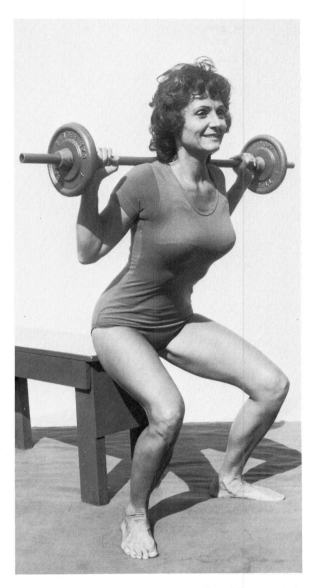

A good way for beginners to get used to doing squats is by limiting the effort to a partial bend, stopping at the level of a high bench or chair.

shoulders to lower the weight much below head level.) As you lower the weight, continue to inhale so that your lungs are full just before the weight reaches the lowest position. Immediately pull the weight back up to the starting point, keeping your arms rigid, either straight or with the same amount of bend throughout.

The pullover is a chest expanding exer-

cise, but it also helps to slim the waistline, especially if you try to pull your abdomen in and breathe high in your chest as you lower the weight. Try doing the exercise with your legs down and also with your knees drawn up (feet close to buttocks) to see which position gives you the best feeling of chest stretching and abdominal tightening. Do ten to 20 pullovers. The amount of weight isn't important in this exercise. It should be kept light to minimize strain on the shoulders, but it needs to be heavy enough so you can feel the stretch of the exercise.

By the time you progress to the point where you can do ten squats with a satisfactory weight, followed by 20 pullovers with a five- to ten-pound weight, are doing 25 sit-ups, and are walking a half-hour or more a day, you should be able to see some improvement in the mirror and on the scale. And you should be feeling much better. This is the time to get into the general basic workout. Work your way into the basic exercise routine gradually, beginning with repetitions and weights you can handle easily. And keep up the walking program.

Once you have followed the basic exercise routine and walking program for a year, you may find that you have reached a satisfactory stage, with your weight about where you want it and that you have no special figure problems. At that point, you can probably ease off somewhat and may be able to maintain your figure with walking Mondays, Wednesdays, and Fridays along with a weight-training workout on Tuesdays and Thursdays. If you find yourself getting out of shape, however, go back to the routine that produced the best results. Exercise should not dominate your life, but a half hour to an hour of exercise a day is a small price to pay for the improvement in appearance and feeling of well-being that it produces.

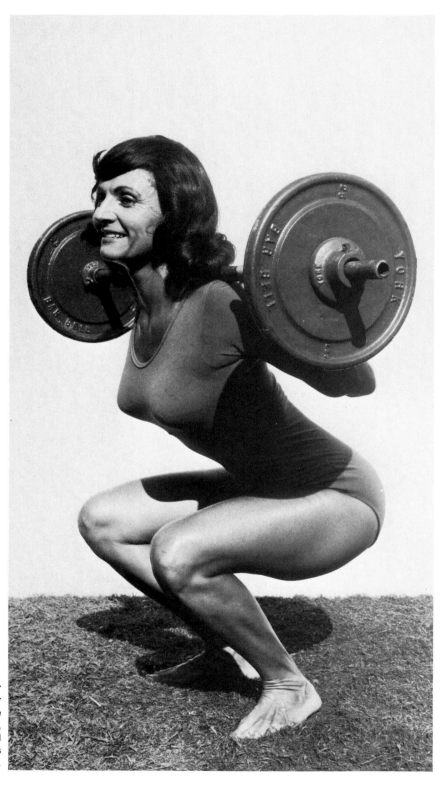

Squats are a great exercise for either forming flabby thighs or gaining solid, shapely curves—the effect depending in part on diet, rest, and other associated activities. Doris Barrilleaux shows perfect position.

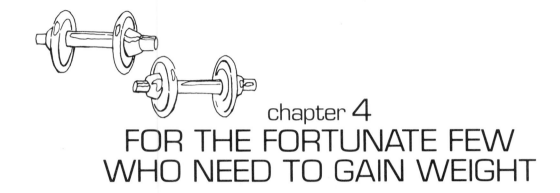

chapter 4
FOR THE FORTUNATE FEW
WHO NEED TO GAIN WEIGHT

With a general emphasis on exercising to keep slim and trim, we sometimes forget that there are people who are so naturally slender that they need to gain weight. Women with this problem are lucky in a way, because they aren't faced with the day-long discipline required by overweight women who must minimize their intake of high-calorie foods and exercise longer and more often. But simply drinking milkshakes and eating ice cream sundaes is not the right way to gain weight!

Just as dieting alone is not the best way to lose excess pounds, so is merely stuffing yourself with high-calorie foods a poor way to gain. In the first place, an overloading of such foods in the absence of exercise is almost certain to affect your cardiovascular system adversely. And in the second place, fat tends to accumulate in unattractive places. To improve shape, which is what gaining weight is really all

about, you need to increase solid size in areas that should be rounded.

Basic exercises are best for weight gaining, and the program should be based on bench presses and squats. See Chapter 1, The Basic Program, for descriptions of how to perform these exercises. For weight gaining, however, the approach to weights and sets is different. Start with the bench press and select a weight you can handle easily for 12 to 15 repetitions. Then increase the weight by ten pounds and press the weight ten to 12 repetitions. Add five more pounds and do three sets of six to eight repetitions. If it feels easy to do eight repetitions, add five more pounds. The idea is to do two warm-up sets of 12 to 15 reps and ten to 12 reps, then three sets with enough weight that it's fairly difficult to complete six to eight repetitions.

After completing a total of from 40 to 50 bench presses in five sets, move on to squats and follow the same regimen of reps, weight increases, and sets. For the first month, don't do any other exercises. Just do bench presses and squats three days a week.

Get plenty of rest and plenty of nourishing food. Don't stuff yourself at three meals a day, but try to eat some nourishing snacks between meals. Be sure to get enough protein, but don't stint on the carbohydrates, either. Your breakfast should include juice or fruit, eggs and toast (or a high protein cereal with milk, if you don't like eggs), and a glass of milk.

If you're hungry at breakfast time, don't hesitate to add bacon or sausage and some home fries, and finish off with a muffin and jelly. If you aren't hungry enough to eat more than the basic breakfast, be sure to have a mid-morning snack. A good one is a peanut butter and jelly sandwich and a glass of milk.

For lunch, be sure to have some protein in the form of a tuna salad, a tuna sandwich, or some other kind of sandwich with meat and/or cheese. Drink a glass of milk or a milkshake.

If you're hungry at mid-afternoon, have another snack and try to include some protein again. Cheese and crackers make a good high-protein, high-calorie snack.

In the evening, eat a portion of meat, poultry, or seafood with a salad and potatoes. Again, have a glass of milk or a milkshake and don't hesitate to have some dessert that you like.

If you're not completely stuffed, indulge in another small snack late in the evening, again trying to include some protein, even if it's only the protein in a glass of milk.

After a month of doing squats and bench presses, and of adequate food intake, you should have begun to gain weight. At this point, you should do one set of every exercise in the basic exercise routine. The only exception to this is that you should continue to do the sets of squats and bench presses as described earlier. In other words, your workout would be as follows:

Sit-ups, 10 to 25 repetitions (hold weight behind your head if it's easy to complete 25).

Semi-stiff-legged dead lift, 10 reps.

Overhead press, barbell or dumbells, 10 repetitions.

Curls, barbell or dumbells, 10 reps.

Triceps extensions, 10 reps.

Twists, 20 reps (10 each way).

Squats, 12 reps, 10 reps, and three sets of 6 to 8, increasing the weight after the first two sets.

Pullover, 10 repetitions.

Straight leg kicks, prone, 15 each leg.

Kicks to the side, 15 each leg.

Bench press, 12 reps, 10 reps, and three sets of 6 to 8, increasing the weight after the first two sets.

Flying exercise, 10 repetitions.

Leg-raise, 10 to 20 repetitions.

Rise-on-toes, 15 to 30 repetitions.

The main reason for including the full range of basic exercises is to assure that as you gain weight, your proportions don't suffer. You will have to be careful not to overdo a weight-gain program. As you stimulate your metabolism with the exercise and pack in the calories at the same time, you could easily tip the scale too far and begin to put on excessive fat. Your mirror will be the best judge of that, but if you find you are gaining too much, cut back on the snacks and step up the exercise with more sit-ups and some walking, cycling, or jogging. Once you achieve the gains you're after, you should do this anyway, for the sake of your health.

Incidentally, if you find yourself at a loss as to what to eat or drink for snacks, you might try one of the liquid weight-gain supplements or make up your own in a blender, as follows: to a large glass of milk, add one raw or slightly boiled egg, half a banana, and a scoop of ice cream. Blend thoroughly. You can also add two tablespoons of a good quality milk-and egg-base protein powder.

As long as you're young and not gaining excessive fat, a weight-gaining pro-gram such as this should not do you any harm. But it obviously is not a healthful regimen. It includes deliberate overeating. So as soon as you can, you should get off it and into a normal, balanced diet.

The weight-gain exercise program is not a good all-purpose, health-building program, either. It includes only size-building exercises and, while on it, you should minimize other energy-expenditure as much as possible. In other words, follow the limited exercise pro-gram, eat, and rest. But overeating and exercising minimally is not good for your general health, so as soon as possible you should add exercise that benefits your cardiovascular system.

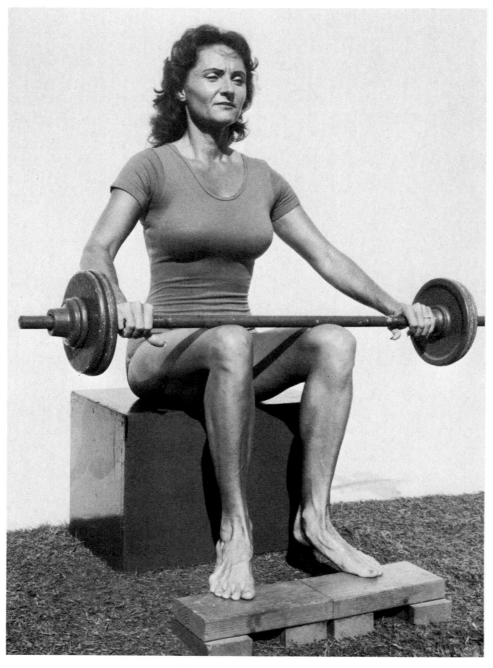

The seated rise-on-toes works the lower calf, but for comfort it's a good idea to pad the barbell handle with a rolled towel or small pillow.

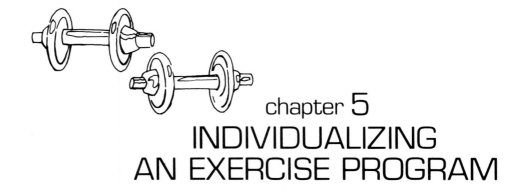

chapter 5
INDIVIDUALIZING
AN EXERCISE PROGRAM

This book represents a solid, general weight-training program, special exercises for common figure problems, and routines designed to overcome both underweight and overweight. As you practice the programs that seem most suitable for your needs, be conscious of your own personal response. No two people are exactly alike, and this truism applies to exercise as well as other aspects of life. To get the best results, you will need to analyze your own needs and also to become aware of how you respond to the various programs, including response to the amount of weight used and number of repetitions and sets.

If you can look into a full-length mirror and determine that you have no special figure problems, an approach such as our general routine will provide muscle toning for figure contouring and the strength aspect of an overall fitness program. If you are satisfied with all aspects of your figure except one or two, you can

simply make small modifications in the general program.

For example, suppose you have two rather common problems that spoil the shapeliness of the legs: hollow inner thighs and calves that lack a full curve from ankle to knee. In that case, you would add two exercises to the basic routine as outlined below:

Warm-up
Sit-ups x 20 to 50
Dead lift x 10, two to three sets
Press x 10, two to three sets
Curl x 10, two to three sets
Triceps extension x 10, one to three sets
Twists x 50 to 100
Squat x 10, two to three sets
 Leg spread with metal sandals,
 10 to 15 reps, three sets
Pullover x 10 to 15, one to three sets
Kicks to back, prone x 15, each leg
Kicks to side x 15, each leg

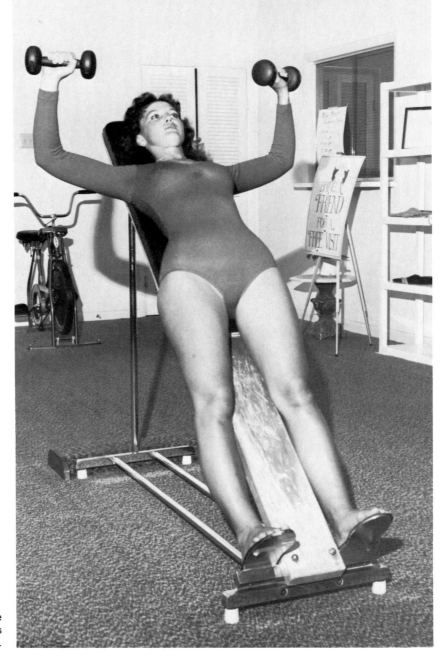

Dumbbell presses on an incline
tone arms and shoulders as well as
the chest area above the bust.

Bench press x 10, two to three sets
Flying exercise x 10, two to three sets
Leg-raise x 20 to 50
Rise-on-toes x 15, three sets
    Seated rise-on-toes x 15, three sets
Aerobic exercise (cycling, walking,
jogging) same day or alternate days

As you can see, the two added exercises
(indented in the outline) are performed
after exercises in the basic program that
work the same muscle groups in slightly
different ways.

For another example, suppose you are
vigorously active in a sport or hobby that
keeps your legs in good shape—such as
bicycling, tennis, or volleyball—but feel
that you need upper torso work. In that
case, you would minimize the leg work

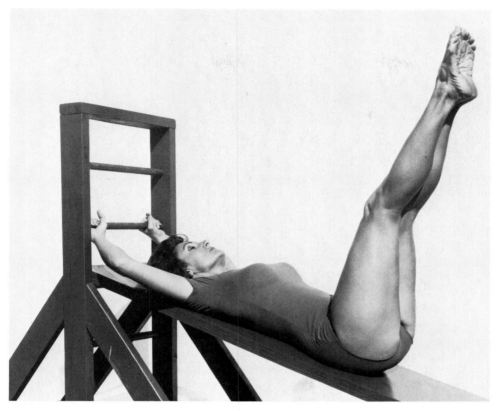

The effectiveness of the leg-raise exercise can be increased by working out on an incline, as shown.

and add exercises for the chest, arms, and back as follows:

> Warm-up
> Sit-ups x 20 to 50
> Forward bends ("good morning") x 10
> Press x 10, two sets
>   Press behind neck x 10, two sets
> Curl x 10, two sets
>   Rowing exercise x 10, two sets
> Triceps extension x 10, two sets
> Twists x 50
> Squat x 10 to 15
> Pullover x 10 to 15, two sets
> Bench press x 10, three sets
> Flying exercise x 10, two sets
> Incline dumbbell press x 10, two sets
> Leg-raise x 20
> Rise-on-toes x 15, two sets

A similar modification can be made in the basic routine as a maintenance program once you get yourself into satisfactory shape and all you want to do is keep in good condition, with all muscles well toned:

> Warm-up
> Sit-ups x 20 to 50
> Forward bend or dead lift x 10
> Press x 10
> Curl x 10
> Twist x 20 to 30
> Squat x 10, two sets
> Pullover x 10 to 15
> Kicks to side x 15, each leg
> Bench press x 10, two sets
> Rise-on-toes x 15, two sets

An abbreviated basic program, as outlined, is plenty to keep you in shape, especially if you do an aerobic exercise such as cycling, walking, rope-skipping, or swimming two or three days a week. In fact, if you are vigorously active in a sport or aerobic activity two or three times a week, you can probably get by on two weight-training workouts.

If you should find yourself slipping in some body part while on a maintenance program it's a simple matter to add exercises at the appropriate point in the routine. Suppose you should find yourself bulging a bit in the lower tummy: go back to doing leg-raises, since the fact that you're slipping indicates sit-ups alone are not doing the job. Suppose your hips begin to show a bit of excess: increase the squats to three sets and add several sets of kicks to the rear, in the prone position, plus more sets of the kicks to the side.

All experienced weight trainers tinker with their routines in this way. A good example is a routine used by Sandra Nista, winner of Miss Western America and Miss Americana titles for combined beauty of face and figure. Sandy is the daughter of Joe Nista, who continued winning bodybuilding trophies after he was 40. Mr. and Mrs. Nista operate a health club, so Sandy and her brother never lacked for either instruction or good examples at home.

Evaluating her own exercise needs after long experience, Sandy developed the following program (as reported by Bill Reynolds in *Muscle Magazine International*):

"Crunches" (a combination half sit-up and half knee-up) x 25, four sets

Leg-raises x 25, four to six sets

Twists x 25, four to six sets

Squat (on machine), 100 lb. x 15, four to six sets

Stiff-leg dead lift, 50 to 65 lb., four to six sets

Lunges x 15, four to six sets (each leg), holding light dumbbells at sides

Lying pulley work (attached to ankle, 25 reps, four to six sets in three directions, each leg (special gym equipment required)

Leg extension, 50 to 80 lb., four to six sets

Leg swings x 25, three to four sets

Kneeling back kicks x 25, three to four sets (These swings and kicks are essentially the same exercises described in Chapter 2 on special exercises for the hips and sides.)

Rise-on-toes, standing, four to six sets of 15 to 25 repetitions

Rise-on-toes, seated, four sets of 25 reps

Flying exercise, 15- to 20-lb. dumbbells, three sets of 15

Pullovers, 15 to 20 lb. x three sets of 15

Pulley crossovers, three sets of 15 (special gym equipment required)

Lat pulls, 45 lb. x three sets of 15 to 20

Back hyperextension x 15, three to four sets

Good-morning exercise, 35 lb. x 25, four sets

Additional light dumbbell work for arm toning (This would be exercises such as curls, presses, and triceps extensions.)

The foregoing exercise program, plus attention to diet and getting seven to eight hours of sleep regularly, enabled Sandy Nista to maintain a weight of 125 pounds at 5 feet 7 inches, with measurements of 36-inch bust, 21-inch waist, and 36-inch hips.

Each individual should strive to develop an effective, personalized program and then stick to it. Using this book as a reference, and critically examining your figure in a mirror, you should be able to add and subtract exercises as needed to keep in the shape you would like to maintain. It isn't necessarily easy to accomplish this, but it definitely is possible. If you give regular exercise a fair trial, the chances are you will come to enjoy it . . . or at least be willing to continue the small investment of time and effort it takes to achieve significant figure improvement and greatly improved feeling of well-being.

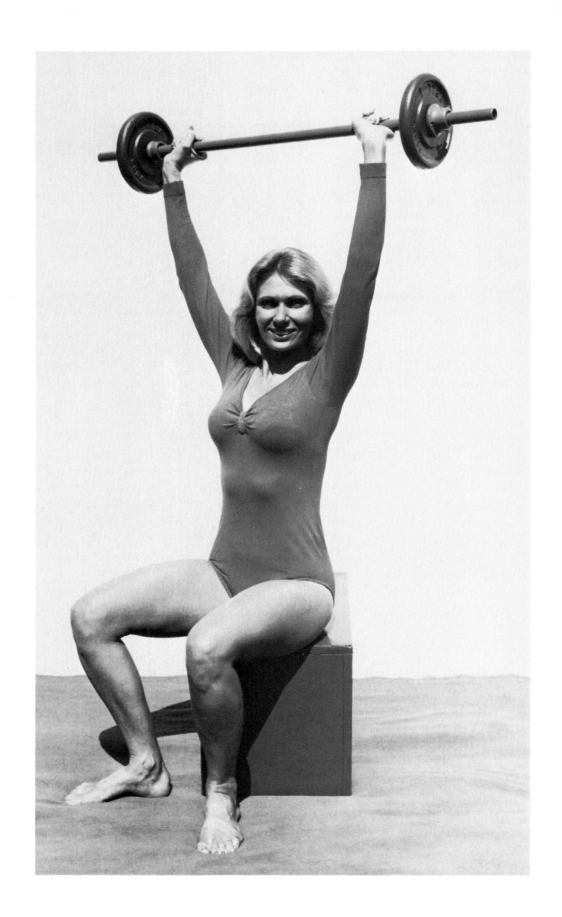

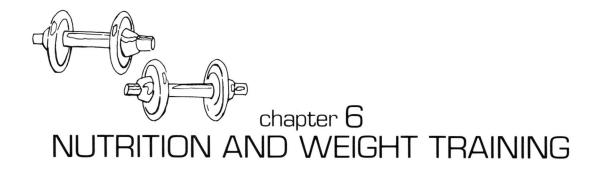

chapter 6
NUTRITION AND WEIGHT TRAINING

Although this is a book about exercise rather than about nutrition, people who are interested in physical fitness find that it is impossible to approach the subject constructively without considering diet. It is certainly advisable to be aware of your body's needs for natural foods and also the possible advantages to be derived from taking food supplements.

Dr. Jean Mayer, an eminent authority on nutrition, divides foods into seven groups that he believes supply all the essential nutrients:

1. Leafy green vegetables and yellow vegetables, for vitamins (especially A, B_2, and folic acid) and minerals.
2. Citrus fruits, tomatoes, raw cabbage, green vegetables, and salad greens, for vitamins (especially C) and roughage.
3. Potatoes and similar root foods as well as fruits for starch, vitamins, and minerals.
4. Milk and milk products such as cheese for calcium and protein.
5. Meat, poultry, fish, eggs, and legumes for protein and minerals.
6. Bread, flour, and cereals (especially whole grain) for energy, vitamins (especially B_6 and, from wheat germ, vitamin E), iron, and minerals.
7. Butter, margarine, and vegetable oil for vitamin A and oil.

Most physical culturists would agree with Dr. Mayer's recommendation that a well-balanced diet of natural foods can be obtained by selecting from his seven groups. In addition, however, many physical culturists believe that the diet should be supplemented with additional protein, vitamins, and minerals.

Concentrated protein supplements are available that are made from milk and egg sources, from animal sources, and from vegetable sources, especially soybeans. Protein from milk, egg, and

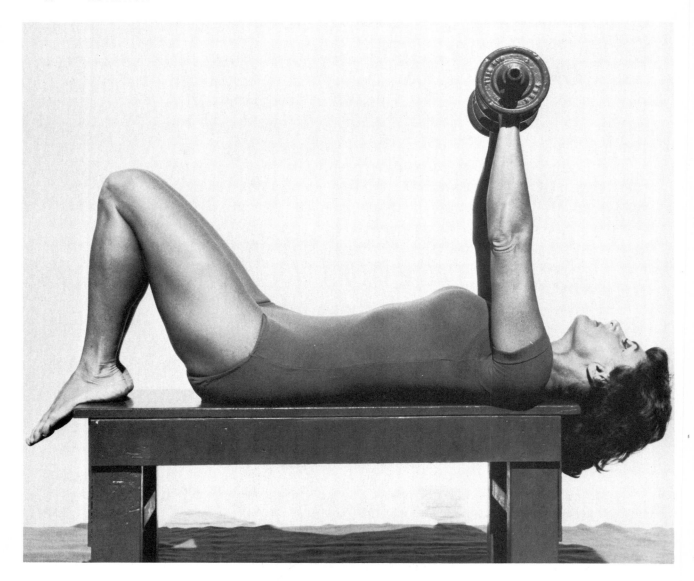

animal sources can be expected to have the most nutritional value per pound because these sources have an amino-acid balance that allows them to be readily assimilated.

Desiccated liver tablets are favored by many physical culturists because they seem to provide energy for exercising and also to promote nitrogen retention.

The most popular vitamin supplement seems to be Vitamin C, which is believed in minimize cold symptoms if not actually prevent colds, and which also is known to prevent excessive fragility of blood vessels. Vitamin C is also essential for strong

body cells, and healthy teeth, gums and bones.

Vitamin E, sometimes in the form of wheat germ or cold-pressed wheat germ oil capsules, is taken in the belief that it enhances endurance and even that it may help preserve youthfulness. This latter belief has not been substantiated in scientific studies, but vitamin E has been shown to produce an effect comparable to slowing aging in test tube experiments. Vitamin E is essential for proper function of red blood cells.

It does seem prudent for anyone who doubts the adequacy of her diet to provide the essential vitamins and minerals to take a multi-vitamin/mineral supplement. As long as excessive amounts of the fat soluble vitamins (especially A and D) are not taken—and most multi-vitamin supplements contain only modest amounts—there is no known harm from the practice.

Dr. Frederick J. Stare, former chairman of nutrition at the Harvard University School of Public Health has stated that "the most important nutritional problem in our country [is] eating and drinking too much and not using up enough of these extra calories in muscular activity—result, obesity."

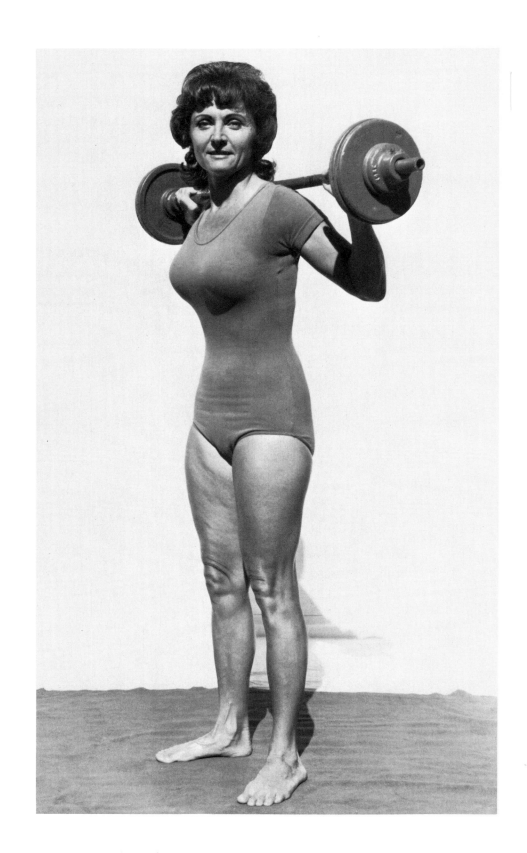

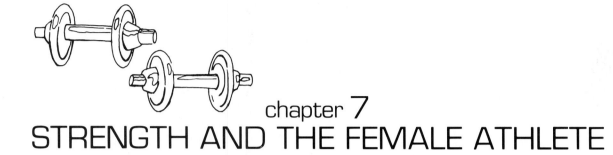

chapter 7
STRENGTH AND THE FEMALE ATHLETE

Just as the benefits of weight training for figure improvement for women were unknown just a few years ago, so was the use of barbells a taboo for women athletes. But no longer. The world's best women athletes in all sports train with weights, and no woman can hope to compete successfully against them without also obtaining the strength-building benefits of barbell and dumbbell exercises.

For example, year after year Jane Frederick qualified as the best all-around female athlete in the United States by winning the pentathlon, a five-event track and field competition that is considered the equivalent of the men's decathlon. Somewhat self-conscious about her naturally broad shoulders, the svelte, 5 foot 11 inch, 157-pound Ms. Frederick need have no fear that any healthy male with 20/20 vision will ever mistake her for a man. She curves where she should curve and tapers to a trim 28-inch waist.

But in action, Jane Frederick performs as well as most men. She has cleared 5 feet 11 inches, her own height, in the high jump. She has leaped 20 feet 11 inches in the long jump, a distance that would be respectable in men's competition in small college track and field. She has run 800 meters in 2:16.5, hurdled 100 meters in 13.24, and put the smaller women's shot (8.8 pounds) 51 feet ¼ inch, to round out her performances in the pentathlon events. Her hurdling is especially good and she set a women's world record of 7.3 seconds for the 60-yard hurdles.

To aid her track and field performance, Jane Frederick practiced strength training exercises with weights, achieving a personal best of 205 pounds in the supine press on bench. This doesn't threaten top-line male weight lifters, wrestlers, field-event men, or football players, but it's an eminently respectable feat for anyone, male or female, to bench press 200 pounds, especially when that lift is 40-some pounds more than one's own weight.

Ms. Frederick isn't the only prominent

female track and field athlete to handle respectable poundages on the barbell. Two others, cast in the same tall, trim mold, are Kathy Schmidt—who set a world record of 227 feet, 5 inches, throwing the women's javelin (1 1/3 pounds; the men's javelin weighs 1 ¾ pounds)—and Jan Svendsen, a leading U.S. discus thrower and shot putter. Ms. Schmidt, towering 6 feet 1 inch and weighing a surprising 175 pounds, could do squats as an exercise with 260 pounds and was strong enough to dead lift 400. Ms. Svendsen could power clean well over her own weight, reaching a personal best of 205—a weight that would challenge most men her size and would stop an appreciable number of them cold!

There is no doubt that women can acquire considerable strength with weight training. But for the same reason that they don't build muscles that make them look like men—lack of male hormones—they fall far short of matching the strength of really strong men. Women especially fall short of matching men's strength in the upper body and the arms and shoulders. Impressive as Jane Frederick's 205-pound bench press is, it is more than 100 pounds less than a male middleweight lifter would handle in a major championship.

A number of women have competed in weight lifting with men, however, especially in power lift meets where the squat, bench press, and dead lift are contested. Sometimes, in the smaller classes where few men or perhaps young boys are entered, they do well enough to place among the first three. (The first three places win trophies or medals.) But in these meets, the women generally have trouble bench pressing barbells equal to their own weight.

For example, a leading woman lifter, Shirley Patterson, competing in the 114-pound class, was able to bench press a

barbell slighter heavier than her own weight, 115 pounds. She did relatively better in the squat, with 160, and approximately doubled her weight in the dead lift, with 225. Ms. Patterson is very strong, though it is true that, as an instructor in a health club, she emphasized exercise for appearance more than strength, and her performance indicates the strength possibilities for a trim, attractive woman of approximately "average" size rather than a power-lifting specialist.

Some naturally larger, very athletic women—such as the track and field stars previously mentioned—have developed even more strength. One who has is Cindy Wyatt Reinhoudt, also a field events champion and wife of Don Reinhoudt, a world power lift champion. Cindy, competing in the 165-pound class, officially bench pressed 210 pounds and was reported to have bench pressed 225 unofficially. Her friend Jan Todd, also married to a former power lifting champ, Terry Todd, couldn't equal Cindy's bench press, but came closer to matching the leg and back strength of strong men than any other active woman weight lifter.

In the bench press, Jan Todd hoisted 176 pounds—a good lift but not exceptional in view of the fact that she had deliberately beefed up her naturally large frame by more than 25 pounds to attempt records at a weight of 197½. Although her bench press was some 20-odd pounds less than body weight, Jan Todd managed a staggering 424 pounds in the squat and 441 pounds in the dead lift! The squat, in particular, would be respectable among men her size, including strong football players. At a lighter weight, 181 pounds, Mrs. Todd bench pressed 175 and actually dead lifted more, 451¼ pounds, but missed a 425 squat after succeeding with 375.

Cindy Reinhoudt also handled impressive poundages in the squat and dead lift, 385 and 375 officially, while weighing in under the 165-pound class limit. Unofficially, she matched Mrs. Todd's best with 425 in the squat, which is especially meritorious in view of her lighter body weight.

Two especially good individual efforts by women were Terry Dillard's squat with 255 pounds while weighing only 114 and a bench press of 226 pounds by Beverly Francis (Her weight at the time was not reported).

Another strong young woman, Ann Turbyne, lifting at a couple of pounds less than the 165 limit, has squatted with 320, bench pressed 180, and dead lifted 410. While still in her teens, Ann Turbyne, who is 5 feet 7 inches tall, set a record of 52 feet 6½ inches with the 8-pound shot.

Some smaller women have lifted impressive poundages in relation to their size. For example, at the women's power championships of 1977, three competitors bench pressed more than their own weight in the 114-pound class: Sheila Hopkins, the winner, lifted 120; Sue Elwyn lifted 145; and Terry Poston lifted 125. Ms. Hopkins won by squatting with 215 and dead lifting 300 to Ms. Elwyn's 195-245 and Ms. Poston's 210-240. The total on the three lifts determines the winner.

Others who bench pressed more than their weight were 142-pound Rebecca Joubert (145), 155-pound Sherry Waltz (170), and 165-pound Stephanie Moody (180).

A bench press with body weight is certainly a commendable feat of strength, even for a man, but almost any athletic man can reach this level. The fact that women are at a disadvantage by comparison with men in terms of arm and shoulder strength is given emphasis by the fact that these lifts were done at a national championship where 20 of the 27 competitors bench pressed less than they weighed. At the men's national championship the same year, by contrast, all of the competitors bench pressed more than they weighed. The 114-pound winner bench pressed 264½, the 165-pound winner bench pressed 347, and the 198-pound winner bench pressed 507! Incidentally, the 198-pound winner, Larry Pacifico, also squatted with 694½ and dead lifted 705¼. These comparisons are not intended to disparage the excellent efforts of the women weight lifters, but merely to point out the biological limitations. A strong woman may become stronger than a weak or average man, but physiological differences make it impossible for her to match the strength of a really strong man of her size.

Where women are at a particular disadvantage by comparison with men is in lifting weights overhead. They just don't develop the upper torso, arm, and shoulder strength to match male lifters. The best overhead lift ever done by a woman is believed to be a jerk with 264½ pounds by 5 foot 11 inch, 209-pound circus strongwoman Katie Sandwina. This is an exceptional feat of strength, but a good hundred pounds less than her contemporary male lifters of the early 1900s and some 200 pounds less than is lifted by the better male lifters of her size today.

Sandwina, whose family name was Brumbach, is sometimes credited with a clean and jerk of 286½ pounds, but strength historian David P. Willoughby asserts, on a basis of thorough research, that if she did ever lift that much overhead, she almost certainly raised the barbell to shoulder height in two movements before jerking it. The two-movements-to-the-shoulders lift was called a "continental" and is the style Sandwina used to raise the 264½ Willoughby credits her with in his book *The Super Athletes*.

The best clean and jerk on record by a

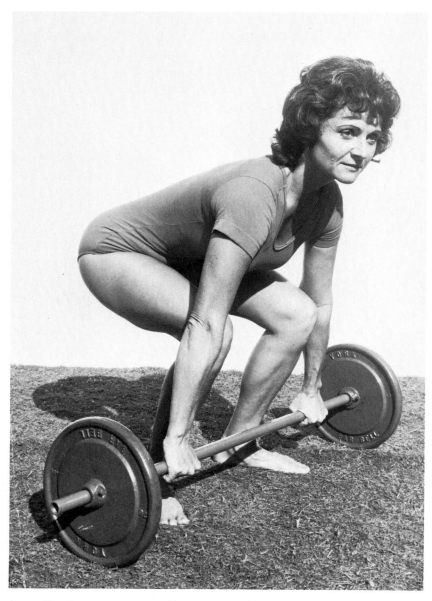

Doris Barrilleaux shows the correct starting position for cleaning a barbell from the floor. This is the right way to get set for lifting any heavy object, with knees bent and back either flat or slightly arched.

woman is 223 pounds by Ann Turbyne. This is an excellent effort for her body weight. Another noteworthy jerk overhead (taking the weight at shoulder level, not cleaning it) was a 230-pound lift by Cindy Wyatt Reinhoudt, done at a body weight of only 155.

It seems likely that some of the husky European shot putters and discus throwers, women about the size of Katie Sandwina, could jerk heavy weights overhead and probably also could register outstanding marks in the bench press. This is postulated on a basis of the fact that they are larger and can put the shot 60 to 70 feet, some 10 to 20 feet farther than Cindy Reinhoudt and Ann Turbyne have thrown.

As the poundages handled by the women athletes suggest, it is possible for women who want to excel in sports to train with heavy weights in the same exercises used by men. The key strength-and power-building movements are:

The barbell clean (power clean)
Supine press on bench (bench press)
Knee bend (squat)
Overhead press
Curl
Rowing motion exercise
Dead-weight lift

With the exception of the power clean, these exercises were described in Chapter 1, The Basic Program, and Chapter 2, Special Problems. The power clean is done as follows: stand close to the barbell that you are going to lift. You should be so close that you can see your toes projecting past the bar as you look down. Place your feet a comfortable distance apart—about hip-width, with toes pointing slightly outward. Crouch and grasp the barbell with an overhand grip, spacing your hands slightly wider than shoulder-width. Flatten your back and bend your legs enough so that your hips are lower than your shoulders, keeping your arms straight. Lift the weight by beginning to straighten your legs. While you straighten your legs, keep your back flat or slightly arched (the opposite of rounded) as the barbell rises. Do not pull with your arms until the barbell has passed knee height. At that point, try to bring it back close to your thighs and pull hard with your arms, continuing to straighten your legs forcefully, keeping your elbows up until the barbell is chest high. As the barbell reaches chest height, quickly bring your elbows down under the weight and forward, to catch the barbell across your upper chest and the fronts of your shoulders. Bend your knees, allowing your legs to act as shock absorbers as the barbell reaches your chest.

Lower the weight under control, keeping your back flat or arched, and repeat the clean either from the floor, just above the knees, or just below the knees. (When you don't touch the barbell to the floor, it's called lifting from the "hang.")

The power clean should be done five repetitions with weights that are easy to lift that many times, and then you should add weight and reduce the repetitions to three and two, and finally do some single lifts. For example, you might do five repetitions with 50 pounds, three with 60, three with 70, two with 80, one with 90, and one with 100.

When training for strength and power, all the exercises should be done in a similar manner, starting with five repetitions using relatively light weights and reducing the repetitions while simultaneously increasing the amount of weight. If you do undertake this type of strength-building program it's important to ease off periodically to handle weights that are only 60 to 80 percent of your best exercise poundages. If you continue going to your limit lift at every workout, even though you are training three days a week rather than daily, you will find yourself going "stale" and will lose both enthusiasm and strength. A better approach is to work to about 80 percent one day, 60 to 70 percent the next workout, and then go to 100 percent the third workout of the week.

For more detailed information on strength training for athletes, read *Inside Weight Lifting and Weight Training* by Jim Murray (Contemporary Books, Inc.).

Incidentally, with all the information we've presented on exceptional strength feats by women athletes, it is important to understand that very heavy weight training is not necessary to produce good results for women in sports that do not require great power. For example, tennis champion Billie Jean King followed a program that included curls with 20 pounds, pulls on the lat machine with 40 pounds, back hyperextensions without

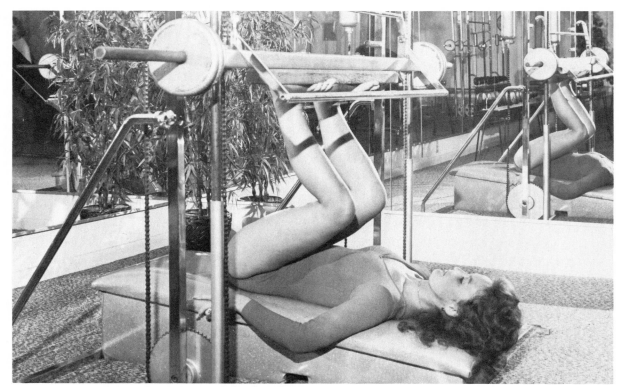

The leg press, demonstrated by Cindy Henning at Hector's and Elisa's beautifully equipped gym in Tampa, is one of the best exercises for the thighs.

added weight, bench presses with 40 pounds, the rise-on-toes with 120 pounds, and the leg press with 120 pounds. These exercises were done three sets of 15 repetitions. Her program also included stretching exercises, running and jogging, and pedaling a stationary bicycle against resistance. The program was well de-signed for tennis conditioning and the weights used were adequate for a sport that puts more emphasis on skill, endurance, and mobility than on strength.

For most women who participate in sports for recreation, the exercises recommended in our basic chapter will provide all the strength that is needed.

A

Abdomen exercises, 1–3, 13–15, 25–27
Ankle weights, 20
Apparatus, 20, 35–39, *illus.* 34, 36, 37
Arm exercises, 4–7, 11–12, *illus.* vi

B

Back muscle exercises
   lower, 3–4, 27–28
   upper, 22–25
Barbell padding, 15
Barbell press, 4–5, *illus.* 5
Barrilleaux, Doris, *illus.* vi, 2, 4, 7, 9, 13, 26, 27,
   40, 46, 64
Bench press, 11–12, 47–48, *illus.* 13
   incline, 21–22, *illus.* 23, 52
Bent-arm lateral raise. *See* Flying exercise
Bent-knee sit-ups. *See* Sit-ups
Biceps exercises, 5–6
Bicycle exerciser, 15, *illus.* 17
Bruce, George, viii
Bust exercises, 12–13, 21–22, 35

C

Calves exercises, 15, 19
Cardiovascular fitness, 15, *illus.* 17
Carpenter, Linda, *illus.* x, 9, 14, 18
Chabot, Amedee, viii
Chest exercises, 10, 11–13
Chin exercises, 33, *illus.* 33
Clean and jerk, 63–64
Court, Margaret, vii
Cross-leg swing, 30
Curls, 5–6, *illus.* vi, 6

D

Dead lift, 3, *illus.* 4
Desiccated liver, 58
Diet, 41, 42, 48, 57–59
Dillard, Terry, 63
Double-chin exercise, 33
Dowager's hump, 22
Dumbbell press, 4–5, *illus.* 6
Dumbbell swing, 1, *illus.* x

E

Ectomorphy, viii
Elwyn, Sue, 63
Endormorphy, viii
Equipment, 20, 35–39, *illus.* 34, 36, 37
Estrogen, vii

F

Face exercises, 33
Female hormones, vii–viii
Flying exercise, 12–13, 35, *illus.* 14, 36
   incline, 22, *illus.* 23
Forward bends, 3–4, *illus.* 3
Francis, Beverly, 63
Frederick, Jane, 61, 62

G

Good-morning exercise, 3–4, *illus.* 3
Gwinup, Grant, 41–42
Gymnasiums, 35–39

H

Head rotation exercise, 33, *illus.* 33, 34
Health clubs, 35–39
Health Letter, The, viii
Health shoes, 11, 20, 21
Henning, Cindy, *illus.* 27, 35, 38, 66
Hip exercises, 10–11, 28–30
Hopkins, Sheila, 63
Hormones, vii, viii, 62
Hyperextensions, 4, 27–28, *illus.* 27
Hyperventilation, 10

I

Incline bench press, 21–22, *illus.* 23, 52
Iron boots, 11, 20, 21
Iron Man Barbell Company, 20
Iron Man magazine, ix

J

Jogging, 15, *illus.* 17
Joubert, Rebecca, 63

K

Keys, Ancel, viii
Kicks, 10–11, 30, *illus.* 11, 12
King, Billie Jean, 65
Knee bends. *See* Squats
Knee injury rehabilitation, 21
Kneeling kicks, 28, *illus.* 29
Knees-up exercise, 25–27, *illus.* 26

L

Lamb, Dr. Lawrence E., viii
Latissimus muscle exercises, 22–25
Lat machine, 24, 35, *illus.* 34
Lat pulls, 24
Leg-curling apparatus, 20, *illus.* 36
Leg curls, 20–21, *illus.* 21, 36
Leg exercises, 19–21
    calves, 15, 19
    thighs, 8–10, 10–11, 20–21, 30
Leg extensions, 21, *illus.* 22, 35
Leg kicks, 10–11, 30, *illus.* 11, 12
Leg press, *illus.* 66
Leg raise exercise, 13–15, 54, *illus.* 14, 53
Leg-spread exercise, 20, *illus.* 20
Leto, Anne, *illus.* vi, 25, 34
Louise, Tina, vii
Lower back exercises, 3–4, 27–28
Lunge, 30, *illus.* 32
Lurie Barbell Company, 20

M

Magazines, weight training, ix
Mayer, Dr. Jean, 57
Metal health sandals, 11, 20, 21
Mental attitude, 33–35
Mesomorphy, viii
Miss USA, viii
Monroe, Marilyn, vii
Moody, Stephanie, 63
Muscle Builder/Power magazine, ix
Muscle Digest magazine, ix
Muscle Magazine International, ix
Muscle Training Illustrated magazine, ix
Muscular Development magazine, ix

N

Neck exercises, 33, *illus.* 33
Nelson, Paulette, viii
Nista, Sandra, 54–55

O

Obesity, viii, 59
Overweight problems, 41–45

P

Pacifico, Larry, 63
Patterson, Shirley, 62
Pectoral muscle exercises, 11–13, 21–22
Periodicals, weight training, ix
Poston, Terry, 63
Posture exercises, 10
Power clean, 65
Press behind neck, 24, *illus.* 24, 25
Press overhead, 4–5, *illus.* 5, 6
Protein, 57–58
Pullovers, 10, 44–45, *illus.* 10

R

Reinhoudt, Cindy Wyatt, 62–63, 64
Rise-on-toes exercise, 15, *illus.* 15, 16
    seated, 19, *illus.* 18, 50
Rope-skipping, 15, *illus.* 17
Rowing exercise, 23–24, *illus.* 24
    upright, 25, *illus.* 26

S

Sandwina, Katie, 63, 64
Schmidt, Kathy, 62
Shoulder exercises, 11–12
Shrugging exercise, 25, *illus.* 25
Side kicks, 10–11, 30, *illus.* 11, 12

Side torso exercises, 7–8, 28-30
Sit-ups, 1–3, 28, 42–44, *illus.* 2, 43
Squats, 8–10, 44, 45, 48, *illus.* 9, 37, 45, 46
Stare, Dr. Frederick J., 59
Stiff-legged dead lift, 3, *illus.* 4
Straight-leg kicks, 10–11, 30, *illus.* 11, 12
Strength, viii
Strength & Health magazine, ix
Supine press, 11–12, *illus.* 13
Svendsen, Jan, 62

T

Testosterone, vii
Thigh curl exercise. *See* Leg curl
Thigh exercises, 8–10, 10–11 20–21, 30
Tindall, Marilyn, viii
Todd, Jan, 62
Toe touch, 28–30, *illus.* 30, 31, 32
Track and field, 61–62
Trapezius muscle exercises, 22–25
Triceps extension, 7, *illus.* 7
Turbyne, Ann, 63, 64
Twisting toe-touch exercise, 28–30, *illus.* 30,
Twists, 7–8, *illus.* 8

U

Underweight problems, 47–49

V

Vitamins, 58–59

W

Waist exercises, 7–8
Walking exercise, 41–42, 44, 45, *illus.* 40
Waltz, Sherry, 63
Warm-ups, 1
Weider Barbell Company, 11, 20
Weighted sandals, 11, 20, 21
Weight problems. *See* Overweight;
    Underweight
Weir, Joyce, *illus.* 5, 16, 34, 38, 40
Willoughby, David P., 63
Wilmore, Jack, vii

Y

York Barbell Company, 11, 20